T0309467

SEARCHING
FOR THE BEST
MEDICINE

The
Life and Times of a
Doctor and
Patient

SEARCHING
FOR THE BEST
MEDICINE

The
Life and Times of a
Doctor and
Patient

Arthur Bank, M.D.

Columbia University, USA

World Scientific

NEW JERSEY · LONDON · SINGAPORE · BEIJING · SHANGHAI · HONG KONG · TAIPEI · CHENNAI

Published by

World Scientific Publishing Co. Pte. Ltd.

5 Toh Tuck Link, Singapore 596224

USA office: 27 Warren Street, Suite 401-402, Hackensack, NJ 07601

UK office: 57 Shelton Street, Covent Garden, London WC2H 9HE

Library of Congress Cataloging-in-Publication Data
Bank, Arthur.
    Searching for the best medicine : the life and times of a doctor and patient / Arthur Bank,
Columbia University, USA.
      pages cm
    Includes bibliographical references and index.
    ISBN 978-9814425506 (hardcover : alk. paper)
    1. Bank, Arthur. 2. Physicians--New York--Biography. 3. Medical care--United States--History.
I. Title.
    R154.B164A3 2013
    610.92--dc23
    [B]
                                                        2013002842

British Library Cataloguing-in-Publication Data
A catalogue record for this book is available from the British Library.

Copyright © 2013 by Arthur Bank

All rights reserved.

Typeset by Stallion Press
E-mail: enquiries@stallionpress.com

Printed in Singapore

For my grandchildren

Table of Contents

Prologue

It was a typical cold mid-winter morning in the Bronx in 1945. My father woke me at four AM and we drove down the East River Drive to his pretzel bakery which was located in a dank cellar on the Lower East Side. He mixed flour and water into dough and then we twisted the dough into pretzels and baked them. We talked little if at all. After three and a half hours or so of work, when enough pretzels were produced, I was allowed to leave and take the subway back up to the Bronx and go to school. I was 10 years old. When I wasn't in the bakery or at school, I was minding my little brother at home until my parents came home from work.

These were the main events of my pre-teen and teenage years: working in the pretzel bakery, attending school, and taking care of my brother. I knew from those early days that I had to find another life as soon as possible if the future was to be tolerable. And as a young man in post-war America, I was able to do so. I was able to obtain a first-class education, fall in love, marry and become a parent, and eventually become a successful scientist and physician. Along the way, I was diagnosed with advanced cancer.

This book is about my life as a student, a doctor and a patient over the past 70 years. More broadly, it is a story about education, medical practice, and medical care in America over this time. I write as a grateful beneficiary of the best of all three. As an active participant in these endeavors, I have seen, for better and for worse, dramatic changes during this time span. My understanding of these changes — how things used to be, how they are today, what is different, what remains the same — is to a significant extent a subjective understanding, one that can only be communicated through the prism of my personal experiences.

I have described the people and events in the book as accurately as my memory allows, but patients' names have been changed to ensure privacy. I alone am responsible for any factual errors.

The book has four parts: Part One is the story of my experience with cancer; Part Two is about my education, and training in medicine; Part Three describes my views on the processes involved in the practice of medicine and the training of physicians, as well as my experiences becoming a hematologist and practicing hematology; Part Four addresses the problems of practicing medicine and being a patient in today's world as well as potential solutions to the current crisis in American medicine.

I gratefully thank Natalie Robins and Una Collins for reviewing and editing the manuscript.

PART ONE

The Doctor As Patient

CHAPTER ONE

The Big C

Discovery

It was March 1988. Dr. Jeff Stein said: "Oh damn," and I knew something was terribly wrong. My friend Jeff didn't usually talk much when he was examining me, and he was never excited and had never seemed upset before. I was supposed to be having a routine colonoscopy. It should have been normal. I had no symptoms; no blood in my stool. I was having this test done for no apparent reason, just my vibes. I was about to go on a sabbatical to Paris, and I had the vague feeling, triggered from nowhere I could identify, that if anything was going to go wrong with me physically, it would involve my digestive tract.

Since I was a child, I had been plagued by frequent episodes of diarrhea as a manifestation of everything from experiencing tense life experiences to bad food choices; they never lasted long and I never was really ill. Nothing new had happened recently to alert me to potential trouble. I was completely well in the months before this colonoscopy. I just had this gut feeling that if anything was going to kill me at an early age, it would be colon cancer.

I was a physician, and even in the haze of sedation, when I heard Jeff's words, I knew that he had found something really bad. When the exam was over, he told me I had "a mass, a tumor", and we both knew what that meant: cancer and big trouble. I was still groggy from the anesthesia when he told me.

I was 52, at the peak of my professional career, and I was surprised and scared and stunned. I thought I was going to die of this disease. My wife, my closest friend, came to see me as I waited in the recovery area. I was dazed and shocked by the terrible and unexpected news. I told her as gently as I could that " I have a growth. It is probably cancer." I was clearly upset. I know she suffered as much as I did that first day and throughout my illness, but she remained calm and emotionally supportive. If it weren't for her love and support, there would be no me today.

I was still groggy and stunned when we entered the taxi under the archway at Harkness Pavilion on Fort Washington Avenue, a part of Columbia-Presbyterian Hospital then, to take us back to our apartment in Riverdale. Tears were running down my cheeks and I was leaning on my wife as we were about to start our ride. The cab driver turned around right then, looked at me, and proclaimed with great authority: "Don't worry. You're gonna be all right!" Magically, his words really helped me. I remember them clearly to this day. But I still felt cold and sweaty and weak and helpless and scared. For the first time in my life, I was afraid I was going to die soon.

I moved as if in a fog that week. Two days after the colonoscopy, as head of Columbia University's Department of Genetics and Development's training committee, I had to meet the new student applicants. I did so with as much enthusiasm as I could muster although it was obviously much less than I usually had.

My colonoscopy biopsies came back a few days later and confirmed the diagnosis of colon cancer. I remained in somewhat of a daze, but I knew what I had to do. I had to try to cure this thing as quickly and completely as possible. Otherwise, I would never be happy again.

Surgery and recovery

Dr. Alfred Markowitz did the surgery at Columbia-Presbyterian Medical Center (CPMC) the next week. Even though I had never had much of a personal or medical relationship with him during my long years there, I knew that Dr. Markowitz had the reputation of having "the best hands" at the medical center. And that's what you want in a surgeon when you need an operation — the best hands doing it! Not the best bedside manner or the best ancillary staff, but the best hands. Period.

Surgeons are not generally known for their friendly and sensitive interactions with their patients. Most surgeons are technicians and healers first, and only real people to their patients sometime after that. As it happened, Al Markowitz, although a man of few words, was an unusually compassionate surgeon, and he always made me feel that I was a person as well as a patient.

Although I didn't know it or appreciate it then, he most likely had cured me of my cancer with his surgery, just as Jeff Stein had saved my life with his discovery of my tumor by his expert colonoscopy. The tumor that Jeff Stein had found was on the right side of my colon, at its extreme limit, and almost as far as the colonoscopy tube could go. Jeff's completeness and compulsivity in visualizing my entire colon had saved my life. If the tumor had grown much larger for much longer, it would have invaded my body further and metastasized and eventually I could not have been cured.

The real world of medicine

My hospital, Presbyterian Hospital (now part of New York Presbyterian Hospital) is an outstanding hospital with superb doctors and nurses, and is one of the best hospitals in the world. It has long been associated with Columbia University and is staffed by doctors like me who are either Columbia professors or have Columbia appointments. The complex of Columbia affiliated institutions at 168th Street in Manhattan includes Presbyterian Hospital; a medical school (the College of Physicians and Surgeons); a nursing school and the School of Public Health. The complex used to be called Columbia Presbyterian Medical Center (CPMC). It is now named Columbia University Medical Center. I had already been a physician at CPMC for 28 years at the time I became ill and I had cared for many many sick patients there, but this was my first experience on the other side of the bedrail, in the bed looking out. It was the most trying time of my life.

I was admitted to the hospital the day before the operation, as is usual. My room was on a so-called "VIP floor" in a then private section of the hospital called Harkness Pavilion. But my experience there was far from anything I would consider special. Until I myself became a patient, I never realized as a doctor how bad it was for patients being on the other side of the bedrail.

My first shock came when a Columbia medical student woke me at 3 AM on the day of my surgery to draw my blood for tests that should have been done the day before by him, the surgical house staff doctors, or, better still, a well-trained blood drawing technician. As if that weren't bad enough, it took the student three or four needle sticks before he obtained the blood sample. Ironically, at that time, I was the director of the hematology laboratories at the hospital, and in that capacity, I was responsible for the supervision of the blood drawing technicians. I was not a happy so-called VIP.

I have no memory of the surgery or its immediate aftermath, and I am eternally grateful for that. I never had any significant pain or discomfort at the site of the surgery. For all of that, I felt I had been blessed by God. Opiates are wonderful medicines, and I had enough of them to make me completely comfortable and pain-free. Although I had a long abdominal incision closed with metal clips, I never felt any pain there or in any of the bowel structures that were manipulated.

Despite my lack of pain, what I did have after the surgery were many relatively minor complications, most of which are expected, but which were all new to me as the patient. Most uncomfortably, I had no normal bladder or bowel function post-operatively for 10 days, due to the trauma to my bowel and the pain medicine I required. So I needed a tube in my stomach hooked to a suction device to prevent the buildup of gas and fluid in my gut that wasn't moving anywhere.

Nurses and house staff tried valiantly to make me swallow a stomach tube inserted through my nose, but I kept gagging and choking on the tube. Finally, finally, someone suggested I jiggle a mouthful of a solution containing the anesthetic lidocaine into the back of my throat to suppress my gag reflex so I wouldn't cough out the tube. I had never heard of that maneuver before and had not thought of it myself in my own care. It was a memorable medical moment for me. It worked the first time around. I jiggled the lidocaine solution several additional times whenever I needed the tube re-inserted. This experience taught me how important little things are to patients. It also re-enforced my thinking that you never stop learning new tricks in medicine and patient care even if you have been in the profession for many years.

I also needed a urethral catheter and intravenous infusions. These were much less trouble for me. I also felt little or no control over my body movements or physical activities for the first post-operative 10 days. I felt like a big amorphous lump of flesh and bone. My wife was there helping me almost all day long and into the night, but when she left to go home,

I felt totally helpless, at risk of dying without nursing hands dedicated to me and available whenever I needed something large or small. I needed special nurses to survive.

I needed someone day and night to give me ice chips to prevent the horrible dryness in my mouth; to help me turn when I was uncomfortable; to help me cough and breathe; to check that my stomach tube and urinary catheter were working; to make sure I received my medications when I needed them.

I could do none of these things on my own. Without my wife or the special nurses overnight, I was helpless. The special nurses were expensive and drained most of our family's savings at the time, but I am convinced they were life-saving.

During the first ten days post-operatively, the world was a blur. I was anxious and confused, and slept fitfully, surviving each day only with assistance. I don't remember much from this whole time except that I needed help to do everything.

If it weren't for my wife and special nurses attentive only to me, I might have been too frail to survive my early post-op days. I, like most patients in the'80s, was on a general surgical care floor. Many of the problems I faced with my early post-operative care have been alleviated in recent years by the creation of special post-operative care units and cancer care units in which nurses dedicated to the care of patients like me are concentrated, and in which there is a greater understanding of patients' psychological as well as physical needs, especially when patients are extremely ill.

After my hospitalization, I was much more aware of my own attitudes towards patients and I was more responsive to their problems and requests than I had ever been before. I was always a competent physician in treating patients, and I don't think I was ever unempathetic. After being on the other side of the bedrail, however, I felt I could do much better, and I tried to be more sensitive to patients' needs. I held more hands and asked more about the things that the patient might need.

Visitors and privacy

Decisions about the people we want around us when we are really sick boil down to individual choices. Many people want their entire families around them all the time, tending to all their needs. They welcome any visitors. I certainly needed my doctors, nurses and my wife, but except for my children, who were in their twenties, I wanted nobody else. I did not want any uninvited calls or visitors. The night before my surgery, I had my wife place a "No Visitors" sign on my door and I pulled the telephone cord out of its wall connection. Besides my doctors and nurses and my family, my only other visitors for the first two weeks post-operatively were those who barged in.

One of the latter was the head of one of my departments. He was among the first and most frequent of my uninvited visitors. I know he meant well, but his visits were painful experiences. I felt no emotional bond to him and did not welcome or appreciate his visits. He would sit next to my bed, hold my hand and talk to me. This was all good bedside manner, but meaningless to me personally as the patient. I didn't know or care what he was talking about, and I don't remember a thing he said.

This experience made me I realize that much of what I've said to patients, even when I had the best of intentions and sincerity, may have had no emotional impact. I became more cognizant of the fact that my words and actions at the bedside of patients might be perceived differently than what I intended. We doctors can only do what we think is the right thing, Sometimes we are mistaken. If our actions come from our hearts, then these mistakes can be forgiven.

Dr. Edgar Leifer

I was a mostly dependent and passively reactive patient during my first two weeks in the hospital. I was too weak and sick to be much more than a frail warm body in bed trying to heal. The first event that really stirred me emotionally in a positive way occurred during the end of my second week. I was just dragging myself out of bed, for the first time alone for my first post-operative shower, when my good friend, Dr. Edgar Leifer, came into the room. Ed was a tall, thin, intense-looking man who immediately conveyed his interest and warmth to everyone he met.

He was a doctor's doctor, and was a long-time colleague of mine. As usual, he said matter-of-factly: "Arthur. How're you feeling?" I don't remember how I responded, but I didn't look or feel happy. I was ready for my shower. Then he said words that would echo in my mind for years:

"Look. You have to take care of yourself. Just take care of yourself. Don't worry about anything else. Not your mother [more about that shortly] or your work or anything. Just think about getting better and you will."

He said this in a quiet tone of voice but with such feeling and intensity that I believed him totally. For one of the very few times in my life, I listened to someone else and did what they said, without editing or modifying their suggestions through the prism of my own relatively rigid mind.

I had made medical rounds with Ed Leifer when I was a young medical attending physician on the wards of Presbyterian Hospital. At that time, he taught me lots about clinical medicine and proper bedside manner. I had seen him take care of many patients over the years, and knew of his incredible reputation as a caring physician. But it wasn't until he talked to me in my room that day just before I took my first shower that I saw clearly the power and empathy that can be transmitted simply and directly from a truly caring physician to a patient through a personal relationship. I had not fully appreciated the impact of Ed Leifer's authoritative yet empathetic approach as a physician until I had experienced it very personally.

As well as being a great and admired physician for over 50 years, Dr. Leifer held several administrative positions at Presbyterian Hospital. He retired in 2007. When he died in 2010, I attended his funeral at Temple Emmanuel. He was extolled that day by all his clinical colleagues as a unique and truly great physician. Dr. John LaPook pointed out "the elbow thing." When Dr. Leifer wanted your full attention as a fellow physician, he would walk alongside of you in your direction and put his hand under the back of your elbow and tell you what was on his mind. The story drew a smile from all who knew him. I also learned at his funeral that Dr. Leifer had diagnosed his own pituitary adenoma many years earlier.

In patient care, Leifer had no equal. He always left his ego outside of the patient's room. You knew he was only thinking about his patients. He was also a great teacher and role model, but he trusted nobody else but himself. He insisted on making sure that everything happening to his patients was done exactly as he instructed, no matter how many of the house staff or other doctors were also on the case. He dotted all the "i"s and crossed all the "t"s himself. He was compulsive about everything. He always looked at the x-rays done that day on his patients before going home.

One of the problems today in medicine is that much of care is delegated and shared by many physicians. No single doctor is responsible. Too much shared responsibility leads to no one being the boss. In a patient's care, you need one boss. Leifer had no use for shared responsibility. He was the boss in all of his cases. He also didn't believe in patient advocates. "I'm the patient advocate," he said. I agree. Ed Leifer was a one of a kind physician the likes of whom we may never see again.

I visited him at his home after his retirement from practice. He lived near Columbia College, my alma mater, in Columbia University housing for most of the past half-century, and had lived there alone for several years after the death of his wife. The interior of his apartment was dark, and he seemed to be living a Spartan life. He insisted on making lunch for me at his home despite my efforts to take him to a neighborhood restaurant. He told me he had just moved his car to the other side of the street to comply with alternate side of the street parking regulations in the neighborhood, so it wasn't his frailty that led him to have lunch at home. In any event, we had a sandwich and tea in his modest eat-in kitchen. He seemed somewhat lost without patients to care for.

In his large dining room, the table was covered with papers and folders so we retired to his living room, overlooking the Columbia University campus. We had a good talk in which I told him of the important impact he had in my life, especially when I was hospitalized, and in my mother's care.

The reference to my mother that Dr. Leifer had made on the day he visited me in the hospital came about because of an extraordinary coincidence: during the same week that I was found to have colon cancer, my then 75-year old mother, living in Florida, was also diagnosed with colon cancer, and I was immediately informed. She had her required surgery the same week as I had mine.

During my hospitalization, I had tried to block her problems out of my mind, but it was difficult, because I was her only physician son. Yet it was too much for me to think of both her situation and mine at the same time. Ed Leifer recognized my dilemma and addressed it head on. "You have to take care of yourself," he had said. And indeed I realized he was right. I had to take care of myself first and foremost. His words had helped me immeasurably to deal with my guilt at not being able to take part in my mother's immediate care.

As it happened, my mother recovered well from her surgery in Florida, and Ed Leifer became her physician when she returned to New York. She had his home phone number, as did many of his patients, and she called him whenever she felt the need. She eventually developed metastases, and one recurrence of her colon cancer obstructed her digestive tract. Ordinarily, she would have required a gastrostomy (a tube inserted into her stomach) for feeding. But my mother was insistent that she wanted to continue to enjoy her food orally. She talked Leifer and me into approving an operation to remove her obstruction although we knew that the operation was dangerous and would not prolong her life. Ed Leifer was the kind of doctor who took his patient's wishes most seriously. I don't know many other physicians who would have granted her wish for major surgery in her delicate and incurable medical condition, but in terms of the quality of whatever life she had left, he made the right call. She eventually died at Calvary Hospital, a hospice in the Bronx, one of the most well-run and caring hospital environments I have ever seen.

CHAPTER TWO

Getting Better

Recovery

I finally began to feel much better after two weeks in the hospital, although I suffered one minor setback during that time. I had a pain in my abdomen in the liver area, and the cause was unclear. What had happened? Had my colon stitching sprung a leak? That would have been terrible. Did I have an infection in my abdomen? That would also have been bad news. Thank goodness, neither of these complications had occurred. The cause turned out to be a minor one, a little fluid accumulation in the lining of my intestine that eventually disappeared spontaneously.

To be evaluated for my fluid problem, I was well enough to be transported in a wheelchair to other floors in the hospital for x-rays and other tests to diagnose my condition. Being taken to and from these x-ray and lab areas and waiting and waiting in the halls to have the tests done was a worse experience for me than either my abdominal pain or undergoing the tests.

The hardest part for me was listening to the almost continuous gossiping and small talk among medical staff, and their apparent obliviousness to me, the patient, during the long lonely waiting times in the halls; I realize that some patients may view these interactions between hospital personnel as welcome and even interesting diversions of a sort, but it was very disconcerting to me to be treated as if I weren't there. I would have much preferred quiet.

I tried to minimize these types of experiences for other patients by telling students and house staff and hospital administrators about the problem subsequently. The goals of a hospital and all of its personnel should be focused on taking care of patients. It should not be a social environment for the medical staff, including its doctors, especially not within the presence or earshot of patients. I am certain that all of these individuals would understand this problem if they were patients.

I know many people I admire and trust who swear by their positive hospital experiences, but I've never heard anyone say it was a place to get uninterrupted sleep. By necessity, doctors and nurses have to do their work on their own schedules, and waking and disturbing patients through the day and night is what they do. My own hospital experience strongly reinforced my previous feelings that most of the time spent in the hospital by many patients is not "quality time," time with real emotional and physical benefit to the patient. Hospitalization is clearly required for surgery and its follow-up; for medical conditions requiring intensive nursing care and intravenous medicines; and for close monitoring of certain illnesses. But anything that can be done for a patient as an out-patient or at home should be done there.

Towards the end of my hospital stay, when I was ambulatory and felt better, I tried to escape from my room as much as possible. I used to go to a comfortable airy solarium on the floor as much as possible. I remember occasional happy day-time experiences there talking or playing cards with my sons. At night, I tiptoed out of my room and into the solarium. I stretched out on a couch there and I could see the sky. I slept there as much as I could. I felt free there and I rested on the comfortable couch each night until I was discovered by nurses and sent back to my room. That respite at night in the solarium was heaven!

Learning the truth

During my entire time in the hospital, I never asked my surgeon, Dr. Markowitz, who saw me almost every day, about what he found at surgery. I never inquired about the extent of my cancer or its implications. I was so involved with carrying out the physical acts I needed to survive, and often so calmed and dulled by medication during my first weeks in the hospital, that I never consciously thought about learning what Dr. Markowitz had found. But I clearly was also in denial and didn't want to hear the truth. I was a doctor as well as a patient, and should at least have been interested in whether I was cured or not by the surgery.

Dr. Markowitz finally brought up the subject as I was ready to go home after three weeks of hospitalization. He sat at my bedside and calmly told me what he had found at operation. He said that he had found a larger tumor than he had expected. He drew me a diagram of my colon and the tumor on a spare piece of paper and told me that in addition to a large primary colon tumor, four lymph glands just outside the colon were also positive for tumor, but he emphasized that no tumor was found in any of the lymph glands that he had removed farther from the colon. He thought he had removed all of the tumor. There was no evidence that the tumor had spread to the liver and elsewhere, but one could not be sure. I had a "Duke's C" adenocarcinoma — the "C" indicating involvement of lymph nodes.

I still have his diagram. I reacted passively to the news, and I don't remember being particularly upset by learning the whole truth. In retrospect, however, I must have been unhappy at some level. As a physician, I knew that the more tumor, the worse the prognosis. Any spread to the lymph glands, like I had, increased the possibility that the tumor had also escaped to the liver, and conceivably elsewhere in the body. Lymph node involvement is the first step towards metastases and incurability.

Dr. Markowitz told me that he thought I was cured by the surgery. He told me that the role of chemotherapy was unproven in cases like mine, and he recommended against it. His view was that either he had cured me or he had not, and no further treatment would help. That was his surgeon's view at the time. He may have been right.

Hoping for the best and 5-FU

In fact, my prognosis for long-term survival after surgery for my Duke's C adenocarcinoma of the colon based on the available literature was about 50:50. Of course, that's just a statistic. For each of us, the real prognosis is either100% or 0%. We will either survive a cancer like colon cancer or die from it. Most patients who don't survive long-term with colon cancer die within the first few years of metastases or extensive disease.

Many of my close colleagues in hematology and oncology urged me to start chemotherapy with 5-fluorouracil, the most effective drug at the time, as soon as possible. I didn't know what to do. I read in detail the available published studies on patients treated with 5-FU or nothing post-surgery, and there was clearly little difference in the five-year survival between the two groups. That was my judgment as a scientist and a physician.

However, I was also a patient, and we patients have feelings as well. We tend to believe that either the glass is half-empty or it is half-full. We are either optimists or pessimists. I am an optimist, but I am also very careful and conservative when it comes to making decisions like this. I have always subscribed to the principle that I recommend the same treatment for my patients as I would for myself. In cases like mine, I would always advise the patients to take more treatment for cancer rather than less as long as the potential benefit to risk ratio is favorable, and I thought it was favorable for me in this case. I could possibly be cured by taking 5-FU to kill any remaining cancer cells that surgery had left behind, while I might not be cured without it. That was a compelling rationale to me. And the side effects of 5-FU were tolerable.

With this logic, I felt strongly that taking 5-FU was better than nothing. That was consistent with my general medical philosophy: I usually opted for treatment of my hematology and oncology patients when there was any chance of a significant benefit from treatment in my mind, especially if the side effects of the treatment were not debilitating. I was not the kind of physician who treated only when absolutely necessary and only when there was an incontrovertible rationale. I had always thought and continue to think that it is worth taking risks when there is the potential for significant benefits of treatment.

Doing nothing usually gets you nothing in medicine, although there are clearly times when no treatment is preferable, as in cases of advanced cancer with serious deterioration, especially in elderly patients with no real hope of a meaningful survival. But my case was not one of those. My worst fear was of dying of incurable colon cancer at age 52. I would do anything to try to avoid that possibility. The one side effect of 5-FU that frightened me at the time, however, was a known higher incidence of acute leukemia with treatment. I didn't like that, but I would have to deal with it and take my chances.

I had always favored giving as much care as possible if it can be done safely for my cancer patients, even if there was only a small chance of success. I didn't ever want to feel, as a physician, that I had failed to try to cure a patient with treatment because I was afraid of the side effects of treatment. I never wanted to feel that I hadn't done everything humanly possible to cure them. And I felt the same about myself. And even if 5-FU didn't work and I was already cured surgically, I would never know it, but I would still be happy. But if I had relapsed and knew I would eventually die of my disease and hadn't taken the 5-FU, how would I feel then? At least, if I did relapse, I would know that I had done all I could to cure myself, even if it didn't work. That would be, at the very least, of some solace for me. Not much, but some. I had done all I could for myself.

Dr. Peter Wiernik

My major decision when I left the hospital was where and with whom to receive follow-up care. I had friends in hematology-oncology who would have gladly cared for me at Columbia-Presbyterian but I didn't want to be taken care of there, my home base, just then. Too many people knew me there. It was too close a co-mingling of the personal and professional for me.

I had friends at Memorial Sloan-Kettering who urged me to be treated there. They offered me more intensive treatment with 5-FU than I really wanted, and I didn't want to go to any particular physician there. Instead, I opted for Dr. Peter Wiernik at Montefiore Hospital in the Bronx. Peter was a cancer expert and a friend and associate whom I had known for many years. I had worked with him on clinical trials in cancer and leukemia as part of a national cancer study group (Cancer and Acute Leukemia Group B), and we had had many beers together as well. Also, Montefiore Hospital was convenient to my home in Riverdale.

Choosing Peter as my oncologist was one of the best decisions I have ever made. He was an expert first, but he was also an extremely empathetic and warm physician to me as well as being my friend. As with my feelings for Ed Leifer, I liked and respected Peter immensely. Peter is a big man who usually has a smile on his face, and he always reminded me of a warm cozy teddy bear. He was just what I needed and wanted at the time. When I first went to see Peter, six weeks after my surgery, the first thing he did was hug me tight. I cried, and he kept hugging me until

I stopped crying and then he told me that everything was going to be all right; and I believed him.

He told me I could call him anytime, anyplace. We discussed 5-FU, and he told me that he would give it to me if I wanted him to, but that, as I knew, its value was unproven. He told me he would treat me with a relatively non-toxic regimen of 5-FU, one gram given intravenously once a week in the outpatient clinic. This was in contrast to a more intensive 5-FU regimen with higher doses that was being used at Sloan-Kettering and other hospitals. I decided to have Peter's 5-FU regimen for the next four years, longer than anyone I knew had recommended.

I had no certainty then nor do I now that 5-FU cured me. My attitude was much the same as it had been back in March 1988, when, without a symptom or sign, I decided to have that fateful colonoscopy. At that time, I had had no symptoms or signs of disease. I just felt I needed a colonoscopy. And that colonoscopy and the relatively early discovery of my disease saved my life. In the same way, I felt I needed four years of 5-FU treatment to cure my cancer. In my major decisions, all else being equal, I was always going to go with my instincts. I was not going to stop taking 5-FU until I felt — in my gut — that I was cured.

The oncology nurses in the outpatient clinic at Montefiore were wonderful, and my care at Montefiore was excellent. Every week for the next two years, I drove from Riverdale to Montefiore, a 10 minute drive, and usually spent less than an hour being seen in their Oncology Clinic and getting my 5-FU intravenously. After two years of treatment at Montefiore, I felt comfortable enough to return home to Columbia-Presbyterian for my weekly injections. A relatively new and modern oncology outpatient facility was up and running at the Herbert Irving Pavilion at Columbia-Presbyterian by then. It has panoramic views of the Hudson River, and is a very pleasant and excellent place to receive care. I made good friends there with two nurses, Susan Vogel and Allison Kimberg, both of whom contributed significantly to my improved mental attitude towards my disease and my general sense of well-being.

The 5-FU treatment was not without side effects. For the first 24–48 hours after each treatment, I was nauseated and felt woozy, in a cloud. It was a combination of light-headedness and confusion. All of my senses were dulled and I was weak and tired. For these reasons, I adjusted my work schedule to having one or two slow days of work each week following my 5-FU injections. At first, I took anti-nausea medicine, but after a couple of weeks, I stopped because additional light-headedness from the anti-nausea medicine was more disabling to me than the nausea itself. I just tolerated the nausea. Today, I understand that there are newer more effective anti-nausea medicines without significant side effects.

Besides his medical and emotional support, Peter Wiernik told me one other thing that I remember clearly from my first visit with him: "Don't tell anyone that you have cancer. They will use it against you." I never was sure what to make of that statement, although in retrospect, I think he meant that my illness would make me vulnerable in the eyes of my professional colleagues; that people would think I wasn't going to be as effective as I was previously or live much longer, and, therefore, be dismissive of me. I didn't find that to be generally true.

In fact, even then, in the absence of the internet, e-mails and cell phones, I could do nothing to have my illness kept secret. Without my knowledge or consent, everybody seemed to know. My illness (and maybe my prognosis as well) had been announced at a Department of Medicine meeting while I was still in the hospital. Those were not the days of patient confidentiality, at least not in my case. However, I must say, that despite the widespread use of patient confidentiality today, when something happens in hospitals to certain individuals, word spreads the facts (or fictions) like wildfire through the world of health care professionals.

Attitudes

I had lost 15 pounds after my surgery and I was weak and frail for several months. My wife and I would take frequent walks together to try to build my strength. I held on to her closely for support, both physically and mentally. I didn't swim, my favorite physical activity, for a long while after surgery. A major breakthrough in my recovery was when I was finally able to swim regularly again.

As expected, I experienced a wide range of reactions to my illness from different people, most of which were truly empathetic. Most people in Medicine, my clinical department, and Genetics and Development, my research department, including the students and postdocs and technicians in my lab, were very compassionate and understanding. Dr. Saul Silverstein was a particularly warm colleague and friend at the time and to this day. I also had a pile of written notes from well-wishers, mainly colleagues, some of which truly touched me.

Of course, I also do remember the few hard-hearted attitudes and comments from others regarding my illness. One of my associates, who had significant heart disease, said: " I'd rather have heart disease than colon cancer. At least, they can treat heart disease." That hurt. One or two other comments were more subtle; and one or two others clearly insincere.

I never knew whether my illness ever altered the way others saw me as an active productive scientist and physician. I was, however, very glad that several of my research grants fortuitously had been approved and funded just before I became ill. I sometimes thought, both ruefully and wryly, that I might be one of the few scientists to die during the peak of their career fully funded.

My wife was not spared insensitive comments during my postoperative hospitalization. Doctors' wives are perceived by some doctors to be very knowledgeable about medicine. I don't find this to be generally true, especially if their interests and expertise lie in non-medical fields. One doctor assumed my wife knew a lot about medicine and told her pretty much everything there was to tell, using medical terminology she did not understand. The only thing he failed to tell her was the most important thing: that there was reason to hope I would do well! She thought that what she was being told was that I had a very grim prognosis, that I would probably die soon. Doctors should be more aware of the impact of their words generally, especially when speaking to non-medical family members.

"Cancer" is the most terrifying word a patient or relative can hear without a suitable buffering explanation. When a patient or relative hears the word "cancer" unexpectedly, out of the blue, they often don't hear anything else after that. I never use the word unless I have prefaced it with something like: the patient has "a growth that we can deal with." Then let the patient ask more questions about the nature of the problem.

If the patient says, "Does that mean I have cancer?" my answer would be something like "Yes, but cancer just means an abnormal growth of cells. Yes, you have cancer but it's the kind that we have many ways to treat." I then let the patient ask questions about the problem. "Is it curable?" I answer: "Many times it is curable. It is certainly treatable. We'll just have to wait and see. Do you have any other questions?"

In recent decades, there have been increasing efforts by medical schools to integrate "sensitivity" education — including the development of students' awareness of the impact of doctors' words on patients — into the medical school curriculum. This is all to the good. But whether this education occurs in traditional didactic form or in the form of role-playing exercises, there is always the question of how effective it will be with any individual student, whether "sensitivity" can indeed be taught.

I believe that doctors like Ed Leifer and Al Markowitz with their down-to-earth humanity and impeccable sense of timing and tact are the most effective role models and transmitters of this medical sensitivity to a younger generation of doctors. You know it when you see it — in plain sight, as clear as day — in your medical training years. The fact that some doctors never acquire this sensitivity is as obvious as the differences among individual personalities.

As a physician, you never lie, but you can certainly frame your answers to questions from patients with caution and empathy for the patient and the family. From my own experience, I know that many cancer patients, like me when I was a patient, don't want to know too much too soon or too fast. We can only process a certain amount of information about cancer, a potentially fatal and emotionally devastating disease, at any one time.

Drugs and the future

I never felt any pain from my surgical incision or the surgery itself. I was given adequate pain medication, presumably morphine and Demerol parenterally (by needle) early on to control my pain. I was extremely grateful for this. I think pain is seldom necessary in medicine today. I have always believed in giving acutely ill patients as much pain medicine as is necessary to control their pain, but hopefully without laying the groundwork for long-term addiction.

As I recovered during my hospitalization, I was given the oral narcotic drug Percoset to control my discomfort. I clearly became somewhat psychologically as well as physically dependent on it. I sing its praises.

I took it whenever it was made available to me, whether or not I needed it for physical pain. When I took it, I felt calm and on an even emotional keel in a way I had never felt before. With it, I had no anxiety and none of my usual hyper-reactive emotional responses to little setbacks.

I continued to take Percoset occasionally at home as an anxiety reducer. I rationalized my need for it for six months or so at home before I finally gave it up. I could see that opiate drug dependence and addiction are very enticing alternatives to dealing with some of life's problems without medications.

Discovering God or something like it

I discovered God and religious belief in a new way with my illness. I really hadn't thought much about God in my life until then. I think that while I was healthy, I didn't need God so I didn't think much about Him or Her or It. But when the diagnosis of cancer sunk in to me emotionally, I prayed to God to help me. I wanted God to be good to me. I needed to believe in a force outside of me, a superhuman force which I called God, with mystical powers who could possibly help me; not for sure but possibly. My prayers to God were very self-centered and selfish. It was not a search for the spiritually eternal and for truth but a cry for help.

In addition to luck and my medical treatment and my wife's love and the support of friends, I needed God, whatever that meant, for my morale and to feel that I could survive my illness. Until then, luck and using my brain were the critical ingredients to me in my survival and success. Good medical care and a good mind and attitude helped, but luck, that nebulous ingredient that sometimes makes things happen in our favor, was to me the main player.

God now became a new necessary player. I had always been a Jew who once a year went to the evening Kol Nidre service and the following morning to the Yizkor service for remembering the dead and fasted on Yom Kippur, the holiest Jewish holiday. I went to synagogue and fasted for unknown reasons: perhaps to affirm that I was a Jew, and/or to honor my parents. For whatever reasons, my Yom Kippur appearances were never made because of serious spiritual or emotional belief in God. Nor did I have any belief in the power of organized religion of any kind. But with the diagnosis of a potentially fatal cancer, I needed to believe in the power of things I could not control, and God was added by me then to the power of good luck, although I have no idea of how to quantify the power of either. Belief in God was a crutch I needed and used during my illness.

My belief in the supernatural then and now continues to be vague. I never thought of God as an entity from which I expected a response. Nor did I believe in God as a diety sitting on a throne somewhere. But the universe is infinite and expanding and there are so many remaining mysteries: black holes and dark matter and other unknowns we do not understand out there. I did not want to miss the chance to appeal to forces that I did not understand if they could possibly help me in my time of trouble. Whether and where God and luck exist in the cosmos in any real way or in relation to each other I do not know, but I needed God when I was sick and I still thank God for my survival today. I still often say to myself, "God has been good to me," although I still don't really know what I'm talking about.

Death

For most people, the fear of death is fear of the unknown. I am no exception to that fear, but the more I live, the less anxiety about my own death I feel, as long as my death is as painless as possible. I have no wish to have my life prolonged by machines or medicines if my mind does not continue to function in a reasonable way and my important body functions do not remain intact.

Either you think that life ends with your physical demise or that there is something more. Reincarnation. Our souls in heaven or hell; angels above or devils below. It all depends on your view of God and religion. I see life as I know it ending with my death. Re-incarnation and heaven and hell are interesting to consider, but what I am certain of is that the matter of my body will eventually be used to replenish some other things on the earth, the way volcanic magma builds new land. That is our rebirth. What more can we expect from our human lives?

I am very grateful that I didn't die of my cancer at the relatively young age of 52, and that I haven't been stricken yet with any of the multitude of terrible illnesses I see others suffer, especially with advancing age: Alzheimer's; strokes; heart attacks; neurologic disease. Physical health is so important to my total life experience as it is to all of us that it cannot be overemphasized or undervalued. If I feel well, if I can enjoy a new sunny day and not feel pain or discomfort, that experience is as great as any in my life. And since I really can't control my health to a great extent, I must thank something for it. I call that something God.

As I grow older, I have less fear of disease and death, and more gratitude for the good and wonderful things I have lived to see: my children growing up healthy and strong; and grandchildren, the ultimate generational gift to enjoy.

Reality

With my chances of long-term survival and cure statistically at 50:50, I always felt I had a good chance of being cured of my cancer. Being an optimist, I was comfortable with that level of uncertainty, while others might not be. Many would say 50% is a low percent. I thought it was reasonably high.

I never felt particularly sorry for myself during the course of my illness, from its discovery, until the present day. I had been a very fortunate person with regard to my health as well as everything else in my adult life until then, and felt no self-pity during the four years of my treatment. I was also continuously reassured by my progress, and by Dr. Markowitz's optimism that he had cured me with his surgery. I did not pity myself and ask the question, "Why me?" I was, of course unhappy to have this illness happen to me, but I had seen too many young people, too many children and young adults, suffer from cancer and succumb. I felt in no way special.

Surprisingly, I also was not depressed by my illness, even though I have had a tendency to wide emotional mood swings all of my life. I was somewhat anxious for the first couple of years after the diagnosis, but I was more relaxed and somewhat fatalistic after that. I never took any medicines for either anxiety or depression.

I would either survive or die. Life is very fragile. We all die sooner or later. It's only a matter of when and how. I always knew these were trite phrases, but they were also deeply felt truths I held as a physician. The only important things I could do were to obtain the best medical care, to have as much emotional support as possible and try to be happy. And finally, and most importantly, be lucky. God or his or her equivalent in the universe, had to be good to me. Fate and/or God and/or serendipity had to be on my side.

But I could only bear my own illness with equanimity and optimism if I continued to do well. If the cancer had spread and I thought I would surely die of it, I would almost certainly have been destroyed emotionally. I don't know precisely what I would have done, but I believe I would have been totally devastated.

I don't know how I would feel if an incurable illness happened to me now that I am in my 70s, but I was too young and full of life to accept death at age 52. Despite my general optimism as I left the hospital, I also needed to be sure that I was in control of my own fate if my medical condition deteriorated. To do this, I soon obtained large amounts of secobarbital, a powerful, quick-acting barbiturate, and stowed the pills away in a special place. I felt much less anxious with the barbiturates in hand. I also had a copy of Final Exit by Derek Humphry, a book on suicide, on my bookshelf.

I believe there are two kinds of people in general who deal differently with severe incurable diseases like metastatic cancer. Those who will do anything possible or take any treatment available to prolong their lives, and those who don't want to do all of that. I don't know for sure what I would have done if I had had a relapse and metastatic disease and had no chance of cure. How much palliative chemotherapy would I take? How much further hospitalization would I take and how many side effects would I tolerate? I don't think anyone does until they are faced with their own particular medical hell. But I wanted to be ready for any decision I might make. So I had my secobarbital and my Humphry book.

As it turned out, I was lucky and my cancer never recurred. I had been saved by my instincts, excellent care and serendipity. I had been spared. I recovered fairly easily after my hospitalization. I was still frail and weak, but my brain was working fine, and I resumed my professional activities relatively quickly. Going back to work promptly helped me psychologically to be optimistic and positive. I was a visiting professor at my alma mater, Harvard Medical School, that spring of '88 and attended other conferences during that time as well. Except for days lost by the temporary fugue states induced by the 5-FU, my professional life was back to normal. I was back at work in the laboratory and in the hospital.

The sabbatical in Paris

I went on sabbatical to Paris in October 1988, for 10 weeks instead of an originally planned 3 months. It was a time of immense healing for me. Paris, well, was Paris with all its magic: most of all, its beauty and calm ambience. It is a picturesque city with its gardens of Luxembourg and the Tuilleries; its splendid boulevards; its glorious museums; so many cafes to sit in to enjoy good food and drink, and to watch people; so many little cinemas showing wonderful old or noncommercial films to discover.

My wife and I walked and walked and walked the city from one end to the other. We were out many nights until midnight or after either walking home or taking the Metro after seeing late night movies. We had no anxiety about our personal safety. We were thoroughly enjoying ourselves. Our experiences in Paris that fall taught us to appreciate our life in New York City more when we returned.

During the sabbatical, my job was as a visiting professor at the College de France, a research and teaching institute near the Sorbonne. I was invited to be there by Dr. Francois Gros, a prominent French scientist who became a good friend. I gave two lectures at the College de France, and was a consultant there as well.

We initially lived on the Left Bank for a week or so in an apartment provided by the College; then we had to find our own place to stay. We were fortunate enough to find and rent a roomy one-bedroom apartment at the Place de Vosges for the rest of the time. It took two phone calls to get the apartment. In the first call, I had misunderstood the price because of my defective English translation of the French numbers quinze (15) and cinquante (50); it led me to think the price was too high: 50,000 francs ($10,000 then) per month rather than 15,000 ($3000). When I clarified the numbers in a second phone call, we closed the deal by phone. When we signed a contract a bit later, the French lady who rented the apartment to us told us that she had received a much higher offer after we agreed on a price. But she had committed to us by phone and she kept her word. We were impressed with her ethics, and we really liked the French people we met all through our stay.

Place des Vosges is a grand 17th century square in the Marais section of Paris, near the Bastille and the Rue de Rivoli. It has magnificent arcades surrounding a lovely park. Living at Vingt (20) Place De Vosges was the highlight of our time in Paris. We were on the first floor of the building. We had a very large living room with a fireplace with a bust of Madame Dubarry on the mantel. I spent a lot of time lying on the large sofa in the living room staring at the wood burning in the fireplace and at Madame Dubarry, and just relaxing.

My wife and I enjoyed sitting in the park in the square watching the people and the pigeons; strolling around the square visiting its shops and galleries; and walking from there to other places, down the Rue de Rivoli, across the Seine, all over Paris, and then back home. We soaked up the calmness of Paris and its culture. We especially liked those late night cinemas.

Every week I was in Paris, I received my dose of 5-FU weekly at Salpetriere, a large old well-known hospital which was a short trip away from the Place de Vosges, either by foot or by the Metro. I had a prominent French oncologist, Marise Weil, taking care of me. Each week, my 5-FU was given to me intravenously by an expert assistant to Dr. Weil, after Dr. Weil saw me briefly. I had to buy my 5-FU at a pharmacy nearby and bring it to the hospital. It cost just a few dollars. My medical care at Salpetriere also cost me very little. Again, just a few dollars per visit.

The clinic I went to at the Salpetriere was usually not crowded, although sometimes I had to wait a bit for my injection. My view of the French medical system was that it was excellent. Patients were respected and cared for with little to no hassle. It was essentially one-class care. I waited to receive my 5-FU infusion just like everyone else, first come first served. I was taken in my turn. I have read recently that the French have about the best medical care system in the world (T.R.Reid in "The Healing of America"). They have universal health care and have all of their medical information kept on a computer-chip on a small card; it contains all of the patient's visits, treatments, hospitalizations, fees; their entire medical record. It will be a long time until we in the United States have that kind of care.

In December 1988, we returned to New York and life moved on. With the passage of time, I forgot most of my medical ordeal and almost became the same old work-focused and irascible person I had always been. My illness did, however, put the rest of my life in a new perspective. I reacted less intensely when little things went wrong, when I lost a grant or a good person in the lab, or did not achieve a research goal. These things became much less important to me. I had survived.

Sally

I recently had a sad experience reminding me of my luck in surviving colon cancer. My friend Sally Spence died of her colon cancer in her 50s. Sally had been a graduate student of mine in the late 1970s and was one of the nicest, kindest, most gentle people I have ever met or worked with. I remember going to her apartment in Washington Heights to have grilled cheese sandwiches for lunch with her then. While she was in my lab, her mother had died of colon cancer soon after its discovery due to a complication called intussusception, a condition in which the growing tumor causes bowel obstruction. In Sally's mother's case, it had caused her death. I had lost track of Sally during the '90s and 2000s, but I reconnected with her while writing a book about my scientific career in 2007. She was living in Florida with her husband, Pete. They both loved the ocean and going fishing.

Sadly, she told me then that she had advanced colon cancer. "The tumor is wrapped around my aorta and vena cava and they can't get it all out," she said. We talked every few weeks after that, and I did my best to support her. Although she gradually had to give up her full-time teaching job, she continued to work into 2010 and enjoy life as much as she could. She had had a good response to some new chemotherapy treatment and to Avastin, a newer drug, for a short time the previous year. She actually had a knee replacement to increase her mobility during this respite, and was feeling optimistic. But then the tumor progressed despite chemotherapy. The Avastin and other chemotherapy became ineffective.

I hadn't heard from her for about a month when she called in January 2011 to tell me she was just leaving the hospital for hospice care at home. It was the most heart-breaking conversation I have ever had. She was crying and anxious. "I just was in the hospital twice for pulmonary emboli [blood clots] and had two operations to remove the clots. I can't take it any more, so I'm going home for hospice care. Is that OK?" she asked. I said, "Of course. I agree with you. You have done everything you can. Now it is in God's hands. You just have to rest and take all the medicine you need for pain and to feel comfortable. You need to rest now. I will call you tomorrow. I hope you feel better. I love you. Do you have any other questions for me?" "She said, "No. Thank you, Arthur. I just wanted to hear your voice. I love you too."

We talked again briefly the next day and the next. She was in the haze of morphine by then but calm and conscious. I was as supportive as I could be. The only things I told her were to be as comfortable as possible, relax, and "I love you." She had her family around her at her bedside. Two days later, she passed away. I was very sad.

PART TWO

Growing Up

CHAPTER THREE

In The Beginning

I didn't really think that I would wind up being a physician and scientist as I was growing up. My life has been a gradual positive evolution from a lower middle class kid who always loved school to an upper middle class adult who became a physician and a scientist.

I was born in the Bronx on April 20, 1935. That's Hitler's birthday, as I have often been reminded. The first address I remember was 254 East 165th Street between Grant and Morris Avenues. We lived in a ground floor apartment of an undistinguished tan brick building six stories high. The entrance to our apartment was in the far right hand corner in the rear of a poorly lit lobby. There were mailboxes to the near left of our front door and stairs leading to the upper floors on the far left. It was a very depressing place. One of my first memories is of seeing my mother waiting at the door for my father in 1940 or 1941 after he had gone for his army physical. She kept peeking out the door to see if my father was coming home. When he finally returned, she was relieved to hear that he was 4F and would not be drafted to fight in World War II.

My mother was an effervescent woman with a long nose and a wide smile. She was the youngest of five sisters, and one of seven siblings. As was the norm of the time, only the boys in the family continued their education beyond high school. After graduating from Walton High School in the Bronx, she worked as a secretary. When she married my father, she worked in the pretzel bakery with him. Later, and into her 50s and 60s, she worked for Metropolitan Life, the insurance company, as a supervisor of clerical staff. She was very bright and was adept in knitting and crocheting. She was also a terrific cook.

My mother's father, my grandfather, was a rabbi. When I was 12 or so, I was forced to go to study my Haftorah passage for my Bar Mitzvah with him. I took a bus to Simpson Street in the East Bronx and sat in a squalid dark room in his book-filled apartment and recited my Haftorah, usually without any comments from him. I don't recall him saying two sentences to me in English during the entire time I visited with him and he never gave me a hug, shook hands or even said hello. Nor did he ever teach me a single thing in either English or Hebrew that I remember.

In my mother's family, there were a seemingly endless number of cousins and aunts and uncles, and countless intrigues between various family members. I was told by my mother, for instance, that my aunt Esther's son, Murray, a lawyer, quite a bit older than me, was a snob. My uncle Mac and his children were also not in her favor, although they seemed nice enough to me whenever I met them. The reasons for all of these judgments were never explained to me but were to be taken on faith by me as the absolute truth.

My mother's major activity when we were with her family was to brag about me, and my successes in school, as trivial as they were, especially so early on. This was to some extent a reflection of the similar attitudes of some of her sisters. My Aunt Esther would talk about Murray being so successful at this and that. My Aunt Lily would talk about her twins and how great they were at this and that.

At the few Bar Mitzvahs, weddings and other family gatherings I attended, all I heard from my mother was this endless boasting of my scholastic achievements, trying to make all of her relations feel envious and jealous of her good fortune. "Arthur does (this or that) so well. You should see him" was repeated countless times in my presence at those events. By contrast, I don't remember her ever singing my praises at home. She was often short with me there. I also don't recall my father ever saying anything nice or loving to me.

My mother was very outgoing, always trying to impress people. She was talented in music, and would often sing songs and dance when with family and friends and try to be the life of the party; but, at home, the spark went out. Don't get me wrong, my mother always fed me well, and made sure that I was clean and neat and prepared for school. I always felt physically secure in my childhood but I felt very little real affection or genuine warmth.

Some of my mother's demeanor at home may have been due to my father, a sour, dour, quiet man. It was hard for me to recognize him as the smiling, dandy-looking young man I saw in black and white family photos from the nineteen twenties when he was courting my mother dressed in snappy-looking trousers and jackets popular at the time; he was a handsome fellow. By the time I was old enough to have my own first-hand memories of him, he had become generally depressed and uncommunicative. I never remember a really warm smile or a stroll in the park or doing anything with him just for fun during my childhood. What I do remember are his threats of physical punishment if I didn't listen to him or my mother, which he sometimes made good on.

I'm sure my parents loved me in their own way, and I always knew that I was very important to them. I was important to my mother in terms of her standing with her family and friends. I was important to both of my parents because I assumed so many adult responsibilities as a child. And I was the source of the unconditional love they wanted and needed so badly. And as an adult, I was the provider of whatever their well-being required.

The pretzel bakery

Most of my parents' life and my interactions with them as a child revolved around the family pretzel bakery, really a small factory, they owned downtown on the Lower East Side, in dusty flour-filled basements with stone floors, first at 87 Ludlow Street and then at 108 Norfolk Street. When my father first came to this country from Europe, he worked in the bakeries of his brothers at other locations in New York City. Finally, at about age 35, he acquired his own pretzel factory/bakery, making a relative success of it with my mother's physical and managerial support. He was the main worker and worked very hard, selling large soft salted pretzels wholesale to street peddlers who came to the bakery to pick them up. In the late 1940's, he sold the pretzels for $1.25 to $1.50 per 100, and the peddlers sold them on the streets from pushcarts for 5 to 10 cents apiece.

My father, mother and I were the only people I ever remember who worked in the business. I became an important worker when I was about 10. I worked there 2–4 days a week, and my mother worked on the other days while I took care of my brother, Steven, who was four years younger than me. So I really had other jobs besides school, either baby-sitting my brother or working in the bakery. I worked in the bakery until I graduated from high school.

I was awakened at four AM on days I went to work with my father. We drove from the Bronx, down the Grand Concourse, over the Willis Avenue Bridge into Manhattan and onto the East River Drive in the pitch-black bleak night, silent all the way, to the bakery. The East River Drive remains relatively unchanged to this day, and whenever I travel south on it today as I not infrequently do, I am reminded of the less than happy frequent early morning commutes of my youth.

I hated being awakened in the middle of the night, and being forced to go to work as a young child, but I could do nothing but obey. I felt like a slave. I did, on occasion, fake a stomach ache or a headache, but was only castigated and usually forced to comply when I obviously had nothing physically wrong with me. Since the reserve worker pool was either zero or my mother, I was made to feel terribly guilty if she had to go in my place or my father was left to go alone. Sometimes, even when I really felt sick, I relented and went. I never remember working in the bakery with my mother; someone obviously had to take care of my brother.

Being rudely aroused from sleep in the middle of the night was the worst of it. I never really minded the work in the bakery once I was there and into the routine. The first step in making the large soft pretzels was to prepare the dough by mixing flour and water in a large metal machine. Yeast was added to allow the pretzels to expand while being baked. I still remember my father climbing up to the top of the machine carrying large bags of flour and pails of water, and then breaking the white rectangular cakes of yeast in his hands and adding them in. Neither my mother nor I were ever allowed to make dough. My father was the only one in the family strong enough to carry the bags of flour up to the machine and make the dough.

After the formation of the dough, the machine spewed out nine inch long and one inch in diameter round strips of dough onto a conveyor belt, a long slow-moving horizontal 18" wide roller with a cloth surface. My father and I would stand at the side of the roller, grab individual pieces of dough, and with a single wrist motion twist the dough into its pretzel shape. Then we put the twisted pretzels onto mobile wooden racks. The strips of dough we missed pulling off the conveyor belt were collected and recycled through the machine again.

We could do this routine of grabbing, twisting and stacking at what I thought were astonishing speeds, much like what you see in the fast forward film sequences of Charley Chaplin in Modern Times. Only in our real-life version there was no comedy, just physical work. We could twist thousands of pretzels in a couple of hours.

The next step in the process was to carry the racks of raw twisted pretzels on rollers to a stone pit in the corner of the factory, a pit about three feet in diameter and two feet deep filled with a lye solution. It was my job to toss the raw pretzels into the pit for a few seconds, then scoop them out with a metal strainer, onto an adjacent metal surface. My father then picked them up with gloved hands and placed them on a large wooden spatula. The wet pretzels were covered with coarse salt, and then baked in a very hot wood-fired oven, similar to those used in baking pizza pies today.

The pretzels were checked in the oven, much like pizza today, mainly by eye, my father's eyes, (only he could do this step), and when they were appropriately golden-brown, they were removed from the oven and stored in metal baskets. I was impressed with the uniformly done hot, soft, yet crispy brown, delicious-looking and tasting pretzels that resulted from the process.

I actually didn't mind the repetitive nature of the work required, although it was a kind of drudgery. I think my experience in the pretzel bakery had benefits that carried over to my later work as a scientist. I never minded doing the same physical manipulations over and over again in my scientific experiments in order to produce something of real value in the laboratory. Not that I learned any science working in the pretzel bakery, but I learned to appreciate the process of repetitive work when it has to be done to produce a valued result.

The most pleasant part of my work in the pretzel bakery was going out for breakfast in the early morning after we had produced most of the day's pretzels. I climbed the single flight of wooden stairs from the bakery onto the early morning streets of the Lower East Side. It was usually calm and clear and often the sun was just rising. I walked the block or two to the diner around the corner and sat on a stool at the counter and ordered. I was sometimes the only customer.

Most often, I had soft fresh brown pumpernickel bread and butter with some raw onion, and steaming hot coffee. I relished my feast. I brought some of the same food and drink back to my father. My trip to breakfast, which I remember so well, was my only respite from the several hours of silence I spent driving to work and being with my father in the bakery. The pretzel bakery should have been a perfect setting for me to get to know him and for him to get to know me but I never felt we established any rapport as father and son there or at any other place or time.

I never really appreciated the fact that my parents needed me to work in the pretzel bakery in order to eke out a living to support our family.

Going to school

On school days, I was released from the bakery at about eight AM to take the D train from Delancey Street to the 167th Street stop in the Bronx which was within easy walking distance to school. School was always an absolute blessing and the saving grace in my life — from my first day in kindergarten at PS 35 in the Bronx with Miss McCormack, to the present day as a teacher and student. I don't know all the reasons for my immediate love of school, but I feel it saved my life.

Despite the lack of cultural or intellectual stimulation in my childhood, I was always a top student in school, starting with elementary school. I'm not sure why. Clearly, school was a more interesting place for me than home. I was always a curious kid and school was a place I could learn new things. Homework was one of the few scholarly things I did at home. There were very few books in my home, and I do not remember reading any books for pleasure in my youth.

But I was a sponge in the classroom. I soaked up information and new thoughts and ideas. I paid attention. I don't remember my attention ever being diverted in class by other students or other thoughts. I was never bored. From elementary school through high school, I was much more of a listener, an observer, than an active participant. But I soaked up everything that was taught.

I always felt special in the classroom. Not that I was more special than any other student, but that I was recognized by my teachers as special for myself. I always felt I counted for something as an individual student in the eyes of my teachers. This is the experience I have tried to provide to my students when I became a teacher. The interactions between students and teachers do not have to be individual to be felt. They can be felt in a crowded classroom.

Friends

I didn't have the luxury of much free time during my pre-teen or teen years, although I did have some. I did play stickball in the streets near my house when I could, and I had a bit of a social life, most of which revolved around my cousin Sheila and her friends. My cousin, Sheila, the daughter of my aunt Freida (my mother's sister), and my uncle Willie, was my favorite cousin in my youth and one of my few friends. She was a lively, pretty girl who lived a few blocks north of us on Grant Avenue. I escaped the grimness of my home to her family's apartment, a few blocks away, whenever I could, from the time I was eight and into my teens. Although not much bigger or brighter than our apartment, Sheila's home was a place where I could feel at ease while I talked to Sheila and her friends. Her father Willy was a big, friendly chatty man, a plumber by trade, and her mother, Freida, was also friendly and relaxed. Whether it was Sheila or being away from my parents or both, I still don't know. But I will always remember the relative calm and happiness I felt in Sheila's apartment.

I walked around my neighborhood pretty freely on my own in my youth. I could sit in Joyce Kilmer Park on Grand Concourse a few blocks away, and there was a big playground on Morris Avenue near 167th Street in which I played basketball. My neighborhood was an extremely safe middle-class neighborhood in those days and I never felt anxious walking the streets alone during the day.

Once, however, at about age eleven, I was walking back home from the playground along Morris Avenue when I saw two larger boys taunting a smaller boy by refusing to give him back his basketball. The smaller boy was crying and yelling. I was no hero, but I attempted to intervene, being about the size of the larger boys. They pushed me away and then one of them hit me with his fist and split my lip. I don't think I cried but I did leave the scene very unhappy. I never even threw a punch. It was one of the very few times in my whole life that I had a physical confrontation with anyone. I decided from then on that fighting wasn't worth it. From then on, although I have become angry occasionally, it has been my words that carry all of my venom and never my fists.

I also remember when my mother's friend Sylvia's husband, Al, a big guy with a great smile, took me to Game six of the 1947 World Series and I saw the Dodgers' Al Gionfriddo make the great catch on Yankees' Joe DiMaggio to take away a home run. It was a thrilling experience for me. I wouldn't go to a World Series game again for another 50 years.

Hebrew School

We were Jewish and my mother kept a kosher home although we weren't very religious. The pretzel bakery was often open on Saturdays. We normally went to services on the High Holy Days, rarely on Saturdays, at a synagogue on 163rd and Morris Avenue, close to our apartment. My father once caught me playing ball on Yom Kippur near our house and I think he may have hit me. Some of my most boring hours as a child were spent sitting in the synagogue on Morris Avenue during Yom Kippur and Rosh Hoshanah, and years later, in another synagogue in Middle Village, Queens where we had moved into a small house my parents bought there when I was a teenager. I don't remember my father ever having any friends in either synagogue. He was a lonely man.

I went to Hebrew school at Young Israel of the Concourse, which was on Gerard Avenue off 165th Street almost every weekday afternoon after school from the time I was nine or 10 until my Bar Mitzvah at age 13. It was a half a mile away on the other side of the Concourse. I never knew why I went there. Was it better than the one on Morris Avenue which was closer by? Or cheaper? Why our family did the things we did the way we did them was largely a mystery to me. For example, if we went to visit a relative, I would never know in advance when we were going or why or where we were going. Whether it was going to take fifteen minutes by car to get there or two hours. Everything was a mystery. Nothing was ever explained to me.

I learned how to read Hebrew fluently at the Young Israel Hebrew school, but never learned the meaning in English of what I was reading. That fact is amazing to me, even to this day. I wonder whether that was because the rabbis and teachers at the school didn't know the English translation themselves of what they were reciting, or because they were too lazy to teach it.

In any event, I never learned to speak or understand Hebrew, just to recite it mindlessly in prayers. Nevertheless, I liked going to Hebrew school, as I did all of the schools I attended. It got me out of the house. It was easy for me, and I enjoyed the walk.

Bronx Science

Every school I ever attended was at the time I did so a turning point in my life. Elementary school had given me an excitement and a will to learn. Elementary school also convinced me that I was smart and competent, and, through the teachers, I felt respected and recognized.

I somehow had passed a test in elementary school that qualified me to go to The Bronx High School of Science, one of the top high schools in the United States then and now, with a stellar list of graduates. I do not remember any pressure on me to go there from my parents. Nor do I remember doing anything to prepare for the test. My cruise through elite educational waters began with Bronx Science and was incredibly smooth for me all of my life; much more so than it would probably be for me today. Either there was less competition for positions at top schools then or I was really smart, or both. I was motivated to succeed in general in everything I did, but I certainly was not consciously focused on achieving specific academic goals.

Mostly, I feared failure and what would happen to me if I did not succeed. I always felt I had no safety net, nothing to fall back on if I failed. So I paid attention to everything I did, and did everything as well as I could.

Once I was in Bronx Science I only worked in the pretzel bakery weekend days, days throughout the summer, and school vacation times. Not having to be there in the mornings before school was liberating to me. I had to take a city bus up the Grand Concourse to get to Bronx Science. Taking the bus and walking to and from the school, the annex on Marion Avenue near Fordham Road that I attended first, then, the main building, on Creston Avenue, I attended later, made me feel adventurous and free.

One of the very few encounters in my life with the law occurred while I was a freshman at Bronx Science, walking on 184th Street on my way to the Science annex. I had just bought a firecracker, a highly uncharacteristic act for me, and I was caught by a policeman as I lit it. I was so afraid my parents would find out about it and punish me. Thankfully, the policeman let me go. I never bought or lit a firecracker again.

Another vivid memory of my high school days is that of walking alone on Creston Avenue after school one afternoon and hearing someone shout that Bobby Thomson had homered for the Giants, my favorite baseball team, to win the pennant in 1954.

I was pretty much a loner while at Bronx Science, making only a few friends there. But I loved the school. It was my introduction to smart fellow students and excellent teachers, who would continue to light the way for all of my subsequent academic experiences. The atmosphere as I remember it was always unpressured and enthusiastic. Perfect for learning, although oddly, I don't remember learning much science at Bronx Science. I was much more impressed with what I learned in English and French, and was particularly fascinated by the performances, and they were performances, of really good teachers. Their presentation of material was often mesmerizing.

I especially remember my first French teacher, although for the life of me I cannot remember her name; with her emphasis on the pronunciation of the unique sounds of the French language, she would demonstrate how "u" is pronounced "ooh;" with puckered lips. We practiced and giggled a bit replicating her accents as we recited "Billie, fume tu sur le mur," many times. Billie was pronounced "Beelee." "Beelee, foom too sewer le moor."

I also remember Mr. Shaw, an English teacher. He was the first person I was exposed to who had an English accent. I remember how entranced I was listening to Mr. Shaw discussing literature; Oliver Twist and Booth Tarkington suddenly come to mind. I would sit at my desk transfixed, chin in my hands, absorbing every word he said and every inflection of his voice and accent. It was like watching a great actor on the Broadway stage performing Shakespeare (whom he introduced me to as well), and having an absolutely special front row (or maybe second row) seat to enjoy it all. And this was school, supposedly a drudge for teenagers, but for me it was food for the soul.

I have given talks at Bronx Science on my scientific research a couple of times as an adult, the last on March 24, 2009. The school has relocated to a building further north in the Bronx near Moshulu Parkway, but the atmosphere was still as I remember it, light and academically alive.

The teacher who hosted me, Allison Wheeler, a PhD from Columbia, was lovely and enthusiastic, and the students, far more culturally diverse now than when I attended, were smart and genuinely engaged. During my talk, I could tell that the students were listening to me with interest and were grateful for my coming. Lecturers pick up these kinds of vibes. Good students make for more engaged teachers, and vice versa.

The visit reminded me what a special place Bronx Science is. As I told the principal who honored me by having me sign a "special lecturers" book, Science will always be special because it has special students and special teachers. The key word I would use for the success of the place is "enthusiasm." Learning and teaching are downers for students and teachers unless the students want to learn and the teachers love to teach: whether it's math or science or English or French. Enthusiasm is the key. Without it, learning and teaching can be boring for both the student and the teacher; with it, the whole process is worthwhile for all of the participants involved. I have the feeling we have to get back to that enthusiasm in both teachers and students that seems to have disappeared from most school settings in the United States. It has been crowded out by the importance of test scores to students and teachers, teachers teaching to the tests and the interference of politicians.

For the sake of our young people as well as for the sake of our country, home life in America has to elevate education as the most important thing in a young person's life. It must replace video games, television, all cyber entertainment and cell phones as the dominant and major activity. Increased involvement of parents in the process, at least in their attitudes if not in their actions, is essential; also, respect by teachers and students for one another, and students' respect for themselves, to the extent that these have been diminished over the years, must be restored.

Social life

I did have some social life outside of school while attending high school. I played a lot of pool after school on Gerard Avenue in the shadow of Yankee Stadium with my two friends, Stanley Meyer and Richie Bornstein. Richie was a skinny wise-guy kid with a quick wit. Stan was a blond hulk who could hold his own physically anywhere. He lived on 173rd Street or so just off the Concourse. Richie lived on Gerard Avenue,

I think. They didn't go to Bronx Science, but we hung out together. They were good and reliable friends. I felt comfortable with them.

I also did a few things my parents were unhappy about; for instance I recall once going to a burlesque show in New Jersey. I read about it in the newspaper, and I went by train. I think I went alone. I was never a good liar, and at the dinner table one night, was caught in a lie about my whereabouts during the time I was watching the show.

I continued to visit my cousin Sheila's home in high school. It was there I met my first girlfriend, Janet Ozarow. Janet was my cousin's best friend. She was a very pretty Jewish dark-skinned girl with very wavy hair and she looked exotic to me. I took her to my Bronx High School of Science prom, and I gave her a sweater with my varsity "S," (which I had earned as a manager of sorts for the basketball team), stitched on it. In recent correspondence with Janet via the internet 60 years later, Janet recalled (I didn't) that when my mother heard about what I had done, she told me to take the sweater back from her, and I did. My mother said, "It was too expensive" to give away.

Summertime has always been a special time for me. When I was younger, it was the time I felt most free. My family rented a bungalow in Rockaway every summer, and whenever I could, I would swim and surf in the waves of the Atlantic during the day, and stroll the wide and clean boardwalk at night. There was a jukebox on the boardwalk and sometimes time and space to dance to slow music. I can still remember hearing Nat King Cole singing, and I still know the lyrics to a lot of his songs.

I sometimes met Janet at the pretzel bakery, and my father drove us all out to Rockaway where Janet stayed with Sheila and her family in their little bungalow across the way from ours. Janet recalls the excitement of our holding hands in the front seat of the car, unseen by my father, as he drove. Often, though, my free time, even during the summer, was limited because against my will, I was taken to work in the pretzel bakery early in the morning, and I didn't return home until mid-afternoon.

Still, the summers in Rockaway gave me much pleasure: floating alone beyond the waves in the Atlantic surf; dancing with girls on the board-walk; being with friends. I still swim almost every day and have done so for many years. Swimming always invokes in me the carefree feeling of freedom I was only able to have at the beach in my youth.

CHAPTER FOUR

College Days

In my senior year of high school, I applied to three colleges: City College of New York (CCNY), NYU, and Columbia College. Those were all that I knew about and thought were available to me back then since I would have to live at home. My college adviser at Bronx Science was not too impressed with me even though I was the sixth or seventh highest-ranked student (out of hundreds of bright students) in the class. My family and social background and relative immaturity apparently put me below his radar with regard to any of the top out of town schools then. I myself was too uninformed, unconnected and unsophisticated to think more broadly on my own about college choices. My parents' only interest in my further education was that it wouldn't cost them any money.

I was only 17, very naive and unsophisticated. The few friends I had from my Bronx neighborhood knew even less about colleges than I did. I was still working in the pretzel bakery as much as my parents could collar me into doing so. I was interested in girls and had Sheila Shapiro's social network on Grant Avenue, but they also were not into intellectual pursuits or dreaming about professional careers. College was something I was going to do, but the details of how, when and where were fuzzy at best, and planning for it was non-existent.

I had always been a "stealth" smart student. I never seemed that intelligent. I had few social skills. Nevertheless, when I had an interview at Columbia I obviously clicked. It probably was my academic record that impressed the school. I doubt that it was anything about me as an interviewee. At the interview, I had nothing much to say and no game plan at all.

Attending Columbia College was probably the most transforming experience of my life. My life was radically changed for the better during the years I spent at Columbia College, and I have only happy memories of my four years there. I grew from an immature kid to a relatively mature young adult.

When I was accepted at Columbia College, I knew instinctively that it would change me in ways that other schools might not. That conclusion was not from any literature I read or experience I had or advice I was given. I think I was right. Dramatically so. I would need to earn more money to afford to go there, even with scholarship aid, and even with the relatively low cost of a college education at that time, but I knew in my heart that it was worth it and I would do whatever it took to earn the money to go.

I was going to Columbia College together with some of my Bronx Science classmates. But I was going to make friends there with many more students from different places and different backgrounds.

The academic milieu

The Columbia College Core Curriculum gave me a first-rate education in all liberal arts areas. I took full advantage of the program, taking all of the required humanities and history courses as well as advanced art history and American history courses. I had Mark Van Doren teaching me poetry and English, and James Shenton teaching me American history, professors who not only loved their subjects but seemed to live them as well.

No subject in college was boring to me. I took it on faith that all the courses were being offered for a reason, and I intuitively knew I should listen attentively. I was learning to be the proverbial well-rounded person although that was not a conscious goal. I was learning because I loved it. No shortcuts, no synopses, nothing like Cliff notes. I read every book, every word assigned.

I was in no "study groups" in any subject. I don't even know if there were any such animals back then. Maybe there was less to learn; less to know in those days. In any event, I learned in class and then by myself. I finished Columbia College with life-long interests in so many more subjects than I had ever been exposed to before: classical music; great literature; poetry; painting; all of the arts.

I only took the minimal number of science courses required as a premedical student (a pre-med) at Columbia College, and I was glad. I was not that interested in science at that time, or in learning how to be a scientist or physician. I took two years of chemistry, one year of general chemistry and one of organic chemistry; a year of biology and a year of physics. That was it. My grades were tops in my courses in chemistry and biology, my future loves. College physics was a mystery to me. I just about made it respectably through the required basic college physics course for pre-meds. To this day, I cannot fathom the depths and complexities of abstract mathematical or physical principles. Perhaps this is related to the fact that I have always had problems with spatial relations, or more specifically, in visualizing things in three dimensions. I do manage to follow the physicist, Dr. Brian Greene, on Nova today as he gives me the big picture of our universe, but only because he is such a terrific teacher. He is at Columbia.

Most of my courses were in fairly large lecture halls, although there were also a few smaller sections that allowed for more discussion in class. There was no particular emphasis by my teachers on classroom participation. We could ask questions and there was some discussion, but learning was not as much of a social interaction as it often is pictured today. We were there to learn from the teacher in the classroom, and study on our own outside the classroom: in the library; at home; the dorms. This was quite all right with me. I was always a quiet student. I never felt I had much to add in class.

The exams we took were objective written ones, testing us on what we had learned. Our grades were based on papers we were assigned and our exam scores. No special points were given in our grades for our particular personality traits or classroom participation. I believe the more recent trends towards emphasizing student classroom participation can encourage showboating, wasting time, too seamlessly fitting in with our current fixation with social media, reality television, texting and informing each other constantly of what we are doing, what we are thinking and how we feel, no matter how trivial.

I have had only limited experience teaching high school and college classes although I have given lectures in those settings. My major teaching experience has been teaching medical students and physicians in both small groups and larger lecture halls. I have been told that I am an enthusiastic and clear lecturer. Early in my career I made the typical rookie mistakes of trying to cover too much material in too much detail in the time allotted. I corrected this deficiency, I think, with more experience.

I taught first year medical students the biochemistry of human disease. In their second year, I taught them hematology and pathophysiology in small groups and in lectures. In their clinical years, I taught medical students and physicians on the medical wards and in larger settings as well. I lectured about my research throughout my entire career. I loved teaching. Because I had benefited from so many good teachers in my own life, I always tried my best to continue in their tradition, and to provide positive educational experiences for others.

I think that computers are an extraordinary useful tool in education today, but I do not think they belong in the classroom. They are wonderful educational aids for use at home or in the library or on the grass outside after school: for research; for study; for review. But in the classroom, they are, at best, simply distractions, and, at worst, barriers to the interactive flow between students and teachers. If a student wishes to take notes in class in pen or pencil, that's fine. I always found taking notes incredibly useful as a way to recall important lecture details, and, from a lecturer's point of view, note-taking signals active involvement on the part of the student.

Powerpoint presentations are wonderful teaching aids, and when available to students as paper copies, they make note-taking less critical, but only when they are printed out and distributed prior to lectures. I may be old-fashioned and slow, but I think that it is difficult to follow a previously downloaded Powerpoint presentation that you are seeing on your computer for the first time, while at the same time, listening to what the teacher is saying and/or showing. Obviously, the teacher will be saying or showing more than the mere words of the Powerpoint presentation. If the only words the teacher used were the exact words of the Powerpoint presentation, you wouldn't need to be in class. You can always check the Powerpoint presentation that you have downloaded on your computer later on and study it then. While in class, I think that students should have their computers in their backpacks. This would also prevent them from the temptation to use the computer for any other distracting activity such as checking e-mail or surfing the internet in class.

It's hard to do two things at the same time, in my opinion, especially while learning or taking in what someone is saying. I believe in no distractions. It goes without saying that I think cellphones, iPods, iPads and video games should be banned from classrooms.

Sports

Some of my most important experiences at Columbia were related to my being a reporter on the student newspaper, the Columbia Daily Spectator. From my freshman year on, I was excited to be part of the staff and exposed to students with different attitudes and backgrounds from my own. I could learn from them.

I was constantly busy after school with Spectator. At first, I covered general campus events, usually dull events, like the activities at Earl Hall, the religious center of the campus. I rapidly became a sports writer on the paper. My lifelong love of writing began then. My enthusiasm for sports and my wealth of information about its details were my major attributes useful to the paper. I had always been an ardent New York sports fan. I also could process information quickly and write a rational sports story the first time around.

I had always participated in sports as a child. I played basketball in schoolyards, and at the courts in McCombs Dam Park across from the old Yankee Stadium. I was a fairly good half-court basketball player, and played pickup games in high school, college and medical school. I had been the basketball team manager at Bronx Science. I even tried out for the Columbia College freshman basketball team.

I soon began covering major Columbia sports events in football, baseball, and basketball. I remember exciting first-time trips to other Ivy League campuses and exciting games at Columbia that I wrote about. I was in heaven. I was writing stories that were being published with my byline for the first time. I felt like a somebody for the first time. My ego was definitely being stoked, and my confidence in myself soared.

My most vivid memories of sports while I was at Columbia College involved the rivalry (at least for me) between Columbia and Princeton, especially in basketball and football. Princeton in the 1950s represented (again, at least to me) the rich and powerful and Republican, in contrast to Columbia, which was more diverse and Democratic.

Princeton was dominant over Columbia in almost all of the major sports in those days, especially those dearest to me, basketball and football, and it was relatively rare for us to have a win, especially at Princeton. My fondest memory in sports at Columbia was a night when we, the underdogs, beat the Princeton basketball team in a close game at their gym. I still recall the lead in the first paragraph of my story of the game in Spectator the next day: "The woods were on fire in New Jersey last night…Columbia beat Princeton…" I was very proud of it.

There were many good sports writers on Spectator. Paul Zimmerman was sports editor from the class ahead of me. He became a famous sports writer. Giora Ben Horin and Ray Sherman were the other sports writers I remember from my college class of '56. The staff on the Spectator, including us sports guys, were very collegial. Competition for the editorial board positions as senior editors, was, I thought, very apolitical. I really learned collegiality at Spectator.

In my senior year, Paul Zimmerman appointed me sports editor of Spectator, to my surprise and delight. I spent the year writing many columns about Columbia sports. That was a real source of pride for me, a lot more so than were any of my academic successes. I have always loved writing. I just wish that computers had been available back then so that every edit I needed to make in my writing could be made as easily as it can be done today.

The Spectator offices were in a suite of rooms in John Jay Hall on the campus. Across the hall from Spectator was the Sports Publicity office, a branch of the college administration to publicize sports. There I met Dick Schaap who would become a prominent figure in the sports field.

Being sports editor made me a member of the Spectator editorial board and allowed me to participate in weekly discussions of other areas such as politics, history and the arts, for the content of editorials in the paper. I became more thoughtful about current events and life in general with this exposure, although I was still very unfocused in my own life and basically immature.

I was also the manager of the wrestling team at Columbia. I don't recall exactly why I wanted to be a Columbia wrestling team manager. The sport was new to me, intense, one on one, different, interesting, I guess. I enjoyed travelling with the athletes, and being with them gave me a leg up in writing about wrestling matches for Spectator. But I was definitely a scut work boy on that job, carrying towels and bags and keeping score at matches.

I also worked for all four years in a special concession program run by students at then Baker Field (now Wien Stadium) in which the students controlled the sale of hot dogs and soft drinks at Columbia's home football games. The structure of the program was arranged as a pyramid: fifty freshman students manned the hot dog and drink stands and did the selling around the stadium; ten of these were chosen as sophomores to be assistant managers; five of those then became associate managers as juniors; and two seniors rose to be the top managers. The seniors ordered supplies and controlled the cash. I made it up the ladder as one of the two seniors.

There was lots of money to be made at the football concession if you got to the top as I did. While the underclassmen made a few dollars, the two seniors could make thousands of dollars, big money in those days, for the five home games if all went well: that is, if the weather was good and the fans filled the stands. Ranch Kimball was my co-senior manager. We were looking forward to making some real money. But in the end, we were particularly unlucky. It rained every football Saturday of our senior year, and we wound up with little profit. We were not happy campers.

A social life

Outside of my courses, and my activities on Spectator and the wrestling team, I had relatively little social experience or contacts at Columbia during my first three years there. I was living at home and commuted to school every day from the Bronx.

Then, in my senior year at Columbia, I was named a "John Jay Scholar," and I was awarded a dormitory room in the Columbia College quadrangle, free of charge. In that year, my first year of living completely away from my parents, I finally got to know some of my classmates as close friends.

I visited the dorm room of two of my classmates, Gerry Sturman and Mitch Rabkin, down the hall, almost every night of senior year, just to shoot the breeze. The bull sessions there finally opened my mind to sharing ideas and confiding in others on a personal level. Not being afraid of saying what I thought was new to me. It was an emotional and intellectual emancipation.

CHAPTER FIVE

Decisions, Decisions

I had a big decision to make during my time at Columbia College. What did I want to do next? What did I want to be when I grew up? I was pretty unformed, and uninformed and unadvised about my future at the time, and had just been floating from course to course and year to year with no specific plan. I didn't want to make a career decision too early when I wasn't sure about what I really wanted to do. I see too many young people today who jump to a life-determining career decision before they are emotionally and intellectually ready do so. They are often pressured to do so by their fear of competition and by their parents.

I never consciously went through a logical process of evaluating my career choices and interests until I had to do so late in college. I was too immature and emotionally confused to do so until then and even then. My fallback position up to that time was that I would go to medical school. Once I was at Columbia, my mother pushed me towards a career as a practicing physician, and I was still under her influence while I was in college. She wanted me to become a rich doctor, and I think she always hoped that I would go into private practice well into my professional life.

I don't know any poor doctors. The practice of medicine was and still is, indeed, a secure form of employment financially speaking. It isn't that doctors go into medicine primarily to become wealthy, it's just that the practice of medicine almost certainly guarantees a level of financial security. I have felt very insecure financially for much of my life, and certainly was in college. I never felt I had a financial safety net. I never expected nor did I ever receive any financial support from my family either in my education or later in life, and I knew I needed a steady income for myself to someday raise a family and feel financially secure. A career in medicine could guarantee that.

I loved writing, especially about sports, but I had no confidence in myself, nor any sign of assurance that I could succeed either professionally or financially in a career in that area. I also felt down deep that sports writing did not have the weight and intensity I needed to meet my emotional and intellectual needs, although at the time I wasn't sure exactly what those needs were. Even if I could be a successful sports writer, I wondered, would it satisfy me for the rest of my professional life? It certainly wasn't rocket science. I finally chose to go to medical school although at the time I knew very little about what a life in medicine might be. And a life in science was not even on my radar screen at the time.

Academic medicine and basic scientific research eventually combined to become my personal rocket science and I am overjoyed with the path I chose back then at a time when I really didn't know how it all was going to turn out. As it turned out, I have loved and enjoyed almost every minute of my career.

I was particularly fortunate to have the option to go to medical school when I graduated from college. I was a good science and liberal arts student; I was in Phi Beta Kappa; I had good extra-curricular activities. I was an ideal medical school applicant, although I am not sure I had the scientific background or commitment of today's typical medical school applicant. I did like the idea of helping people, but it was not an overwhelming need or goal. Like most of us, I wanted most to do something I loved to do.

Harvard Med

I had applied to Columbia's medical school, the College of Physicians and Surgeons (P&S), a part of Columbia-Presbyterian Medical Center. I thought I would go there for sure if I were accepted. I was in awe of the reputation of the school and its great stone structures rising from Washington Heights; they were the tallest buildings in northern Manhattan then and remain so today. I would have been delighted to go there. I was pretty sure I would be accepted there with my college record, but it was no sure thing. I also applied to New York University, Yale, Harvard and Cornell medical schools.

I was never interviewed at Yale or Cornell. I never knew why. Harvard invited me for an interview. One sunny day in the fall of 1955, I drove to

Boston in my used 1950 blue Oldsmobile convertible, up the Merritt and Wilbur Cross Parkways. The road was fairly clear but then a car with two young girls in it about my age appeared and passed me. I smiled at the girls as they passed and then I re-passed their car. And so it went. I passed them and they re-passed me. Road flirting: not a good idea.

The police stopped me on the parkway at Wallingford, Connecticut for speeding. The girls' car flew away down the road into the wind. I was directed to follow the police car to the nearest police station. I faced a judge who offered me a choice: go to jail or pay a fine. I paid the fine in cash. It was all of the money I had brought with me, about $50, a lot then. There were no credit cards in those days, and checks were not accepted. I didn't know about speed traps back then, nor am I sure whether Wallingford was indeed a speed trap. What I do remember is that I had to look up some friends in Cambridge when I got there to borrow enough money for the trip home.

At my Harvard Medical School (HMS) interviews, I talked with two interesting people, one at the Dean's office and the other at the Boston City Hospital. The dean's office person, an elderly gray-haired man whose name I forget, asked me why I wanted to go into medicine. I gave him my stock answer: I wanted to help people. He said that a medical career could include many ways of helping people: practicing medicine, doing research, being an administrator, doing public health. I had never thought about all of those choices before.

My other interviewer was a researcher, Dr. Edward Kass, and we met in his BCH laboratory. He was very gentle, kind and solicitous to me. I don't remember what we talked about, but I came away feeling that Harvard Med would be a very warm place to go to school, and that people on the faculty there were really nice. Those impressions proved to be right.

I was working in the main post office in Manhattan over Christmas of 1955 to earn some extra money when I received acceptance letters from Columbia P&S and Harvard Med on the same day. Columbia had been uncharacteristically late in accepting me. I had assumed all along up to that time that I would be staying in New York and going there. Harvard's acceptance letter was a pleasant surprise. I had a choice. I felt very lucky.

I had been in New York all my life, and I wanted to get away from my parents. I would probably have had to live at home if I went to Columbia. Harvard, of course, had a great reputation, not that I knew any of the details, but it would cost me more money to live away from home. But I would find a way. Harvard was offering me a partial scholarship: $600 a year. The total tuition was $1000 a year back then (yes, that's right: $1000). I could work during the summer and during school to earn the rest of the tuition and my room and board. I had a decision to make, but it didn't take me long. I was going to Harvard Medical School.

HMS is located in the Roxbury section of Boston across the Charles River from Harvard College in Cambridge and away from the rest of the university. It has its own grass-covered quadrangle, reminiscent to me of the one at Columbia College, with many impressive stone buildings. In my first year there, 1956, I lived on Avenue Louis Pasteur, at Vanderbilt Hall, the principal dormitory, for men only then, just across from the quadrangle. I rolled out of bed and crossed the street to get to classes. Down the block in the opposite direction was Boston's Boys High School and not far away was the Boston fens and Fenway Park.

The Peter Bent Brigham Hospital, the Beth Israel Hospital, and Boston Children's Hospital, three of the Harvard teaching hospitals were close by. We were also close to Boston University with its many datable college girls; and the trolley on Commonwealth Avenue took one quickly to Symphony Hall.

I had a private room at one end of the fifth floor of Vanderbilt Hall during my freshman year. I hung my Impressionist prints of Van Gogh, Monet and Degas on the walls, made friends and settled in. Classes in anatomy were dominated by cadaver dissection and attention to Gray's Anatomy. I found my first investigations into the structure of the human body to be fascinating and loved the course in gross anatomy. Everything was new to me. I sat and looked at the diagrams in Gray's Anatomy for hours, comparing the blood vessels, nerves, muscles and tissues with what I was seeing in the flesh in my cadaver dissection class. I found the intricacies of the structures of the human body hypnotizing, and realized they were important for me to know as a future physician.

What I found difficult to bear, however, was the smell of formaldehyde, the preservative used for the cadavers. The odor didn't leave me for the whole year. It stuck to my clothes, my nostrils, all of me, it seemed, as I ate or slept. I could not escape it. I also didn't do well when the so-called "man in the pan" sessions were held. These were the smaller class sections in which the organs removed at autopsy from interesting patients, also smelling of formaldehyde, were shown to us, in small groups, up close and personal. I almost fainted at the first of these as the instructor summarized the case and I kept thinking about an intact human being whose organs I was now viewing. I think it was the pelvic organs of a young woman who had died in childbirth. I had to sit down. I did better subsequently when I managed to disconnect my thoughts of the once alive person whose organs were being shown from the appearance of the organs themselves.

Histology, the microscopic study of normal tissues, was another first year subject I remember and enjoyed. I hadn't looked down a microscope much in college biology, and had never been exposed to histology before. We needed our own microscopes for the course to examine our own set of slides. Jordan Cohen, "Jordie" as he was known, was my neighbor on the stool next to me in the class. He was from Yale and had taken a course in histology in college. He also owned a binocular microscope: one with two eyepieces to look through and that was easy to use. And he knew how to use it.

I, on the other hand, was renting an old monocular microscope from HMS, which Jordie taught me how to use. He taught me how to fix the light so I could see the tissue section clearly and how to get the tissue I was looking at into focus; he also helped me learn to identify tissues and structures and to use oil to see tissues at high magnification. He was really nice to me then when we had just met and barely knew each other. I needed his help and he gave it freely. We soon became good friends and remained so for years. He eventually became a prominent renal physician and an important medical spokesman as head of the Association of American Medical Colleges. But I remember him best as the nice guy who guided me in histology when I really needed help.

In my second year, pathology and pharmacology were the most important courses. They were my favorite subjects, and I immersed myself in them and excelled in them. Understanding the pathology of disease is key to pathophysiology, the understanding of how disease develops. It is the basis for the way I think about medical illness: what is its basic pathophysiology? And detailed knowledge of pharmacology is also vital in medicine: knowing drugs and how they work is the basis of almost all medical therapy.

Medicine

HMS had five hospitals where students did their clinical rotations in medicine, surgery, pediatrics, etc. In addition to Children's, the Brigham, and Beth Israel (BI) nearby, there was the Massachusetts General Hospital (MGH) and the Boston City Hospital (BCH). I was assigned my third year medicine rotation, my introduction to clinical medicine, at the BI.

Medicine at the BI was largely a bore to me. I was expecting intensity and excitement there during that rotation, my first exposure to clinical medicine, but they never materialized. I did see patients and learn medicine but it was all pedestrian, unlike my previous HMS academic experiences. At the time, I was really looking forward to specializing in internal medicine. But I was so disappointed with the BI experience that I thought for the first time while I was there that I might not go into internal medicine after all. My attending physicians were generally uninspiring during rounds. The physicians in the doctor's lounge would more likely be talking about their stocks and investments than about medicine or family or anything else.

Medicine in the '50s was financially as well as professionally rewarding for physicians in private practice, and there were doctors who practiced at the Harvard hospitals who were quite rich. Some were well off because of inherited wealth, but others had large private practices that generated extensive money. We medical students were vaguely aware of the variety of medical careers and levels of incomes that could be attained in medicine at that time. It was pretty much the same spectrum as exists for physicians today.

A song in our second year show in 1958, the "Aeschylapian Show," presented by the Aeschylapian Club, an HMS alumni organization, lampooned not only the variety of careers and activities that we were mindful of at the time, but also some of the more cynical attitudes of medical students and physicians of which we were also aware. The song was sung in two parts to the music of the song: "You're Just In Love," from the hit 1950's musical, "Call Me Madam."

(Part one: sung first:)

Research is a great big pack of lies.
Screw your buddy, win the Nobel Prize.
All this crap to help humanity
Just eats my guts,
I'm going nuts.
I owe money on my underwear;
Kids run hungry with their asses bare.
Can't afford a pot to pee in, man;
We tinkle in a can;
We're really beat.

(Part two:)

I'm in this game for money.
Being rich isn't funny.
I'm in love with my bank account.
I split fees with my cousin;
We scrape wombs by the dozen;
Curettage pays my income tax.
I just treat upper classes;
And boy, I kiss their asses,
Then eat lunch at the Harvard Club.
First I treat their failing hearts,
Then review their private parts.
I'm a doc who loves mankind.

(Then repeated with Parts one and two sung together.)

Whenever I lament, as I often do, about how much more money-driven the practice of medicine has become and how competitive medical research has become in recent times, remembering this song reminds me not to idealize the past.

Better medicine

In the fourth year at HMS, I had my medicine course at the Brigham and it was much more emotionally and intellectually satisfying for me. I felt proud to be a budding physician. I saw interesting patients and very sick patients and I felt truly part of the medical team. Maybe this was because I was now a fourth year student and had more experience and could be trusted more. When I came to Columbia and taught at P&S years later, the third year medicine course was the most intensive one for students; maybe at Harvard when I was there, it was fourth year medicine in which students were more intensively involved.

I particularly remember the end of one weekend on duty as a fourth year student at the Brigham. I had gotten little sleep Saturday and Sunday nights, and Monday had also been a busy day in the hospital and I didn't get to leave until after dark that night. It had been a long hard weekend but one of gratifying work. Although I was really tired, I was feeling very proud of myself for the many good deeds I had done in helping so many patients over the weekend.

I had left my old blue Oldsmobile convertible in the Brigham parking lot Saturday morning. When I came out Monday night, I looked and looked for it. It was gone. I mentally groped for explanations for its absence and came up with none. I gave up, reported my loss to the police and went home. Tuesday afternoon I received a telephone call that my car had been found abandoned in the middle of the street in some suburb of Boston. I could pick it up at any time at a car pound. I had to pay a huge fine that I could ill afford to retrieve it.

That event was one of many that taught me never to feel too impressed with myself or my deeds. There's always something bad that can be lurking around the corner to even things out. That's called living. It doesn't mean you can't feel good about yourself at times for doing the right thing for the right reasons. Just don't make too big a deal of it.

Another experience many years later with similar vibes that comes to my mind is my drive from Durango to Albuquerque to catch a plane back home after attending a scientific conference with one of my graduate students at Columbia, Dina Markowitz. We had presented some of our lab's recent findings there on new ways to add genes to cells, which could be used to do safe human gene therapy. We had done well and I felt at the top of my field in research. I was feeling very proud of myself. On the car trip back to the airport through the desert, surrounded by the beautiful red rock mountains, Dina asked me about my achievements in science and I waxed poetic rather expansively about what I had done. Not quite boasting, but close. Five days later, I had the colonoscopy that led to the discovery of my colon cancer.

New friends

While I was a fourth year student at the Brigham, I met Dr. Warren Wacker, an HMS professor, and I participated in a mini-research project of his, measuring an enzyme, lactic dehydrogenase (LDH), as a potential diagnostic test for different kinds of disease in different patients. It wasn't much of a research project in itself, but the personal relationship I established with Dr. Wacker was very important to me. He was my first professional role model. He was a frank and open person as well as a well-respected and knowledgeable clinician, who shared his thoughts with me, a young student, as if I were his friend. The experience rubbed off on me and was one that guided me in many of my future relationships with young people who subsequently worked with me.

As at Columbia College, I found almost all of my fellow students at HMS very collegial. I felt extremely fortunate for that. I do not remember a single substantive bad experience working with any of my fellow medical students during any of my four years there. Of course, there was always some subtle competition to excel, to impress our professors, but it never descended into acrimony.

Maybe the competition is tougher today; maybe the standards are higher; or maybe the positive academic experiences I had didn't reflect the more general atmosphere. I certainly don't know why, but almost all of my educational experiences were extremely pleasant. On the other hand, the experiences I had with some of my competitors in my scientific research activities later in life, are quite another story.

To save money, after living in Vanderbilt Hall during my first year at HMS, I moved to the Free Hospital for Women in Jamaica Plain, a hospital specializing in gynecological disorders, where I was given free room and board for "coding" medical records. My job was to put the appropriate standard numerical codes for specific diagnoses on all of the medical records of patients discharged from the hospital. It was quite a good deal for me. Once I memorized the numerical codes for the common diagnoses like "Complete hysterectomy with bilateral salpingo-oopherectomy," it took me only about two hours a week to earn my room and board.

The private bedrooms students occupied were across the street from the hospital on the top floor of a three-story brick building that housed the offices of Dr. John Rock. Dr. Rock was an eminent gynecologist, who worked on contraceptive pills in their early days. This was the late 1950s. Dr. Rock was a great doctor but was anathema to the Catholic community of which he was a part because of his advocacy of the wider use of contraception. He was a very wise patrician presence in our building, always willing to chat and give advice. A tall handsome white-haired Bostonian, he had an easy laugh and a wry sense of humor.

I had two floor-mates while living at the Free Hospital, Dick McClintock and Jack Buchanan, both classmates at HMS. Buchanan was a real character. He only worked at night and seemed to hardly ever sleep. He was very smart and had a great sense of humor. I was always catching him up on schoolwork that he had missed by sleeping in. McClintock was handsome and a real ladies man. I don't remember what they did to earn their keep. We all got along fine and became good friends. Dr. Rock always had kind words for us, and tolerated the not infrequent visits to our rooms of guests, mostly female. At heart, Dr. Rock was an endearingly conservative man. When our paths crossed the day after I had introduced him to a young woman whom I had recently met and whom less than three years later I would marry, he solemnly asked me what my intentions were.

I had two other jobs besides working at the Free Hospital while at HMS. One was working in the Blood Bank of the MGH, one or two nights a week, whenever I could manage to get a shift, since it paid relatively well, typing and cross-matching blood for transfusions. I didn't get much sleep the nights I stayed there, from eight PM to eight AM. The most memorable and annoying part of that job was how often I would be called at one or two AM and told by a resident physician: "I'm going to call you in a couple of hours to type and cross-match blood on my patient." I always wondered why I received this preliminary call that woke me from sleep hours before I had to do anything, unless it was to make sure someone was on duty. I wondered how they would have felt if I had called them unnecessarily when they were asleep or resting about something that didn't have to be done until hours later.

My other part-time job was as a re-write man in the Sports Department at the Boston Globe. I worked there, again nights, writing up stories about college and pro sports events that The Globe did not cover with live reporters; the reports were relayed to me by telephone by people at the events. I wrote a paragraph or two about each event that was published in the paper the next day. Just the facts. No bylines. I enjoyed that job very much. It reminded me of my college days.

Summers and money

Throughout college and medical school, I always knew that I could do the schoolwork required and anything else I needed to do quickly and easily. But I always needed money to live and survive. I knew my parents would not or could not provide any of it for me to go to college or to medical school, or any time after that either, so I always had to work. My last summer in high school, I worked as a customs runner for a customs clearing firm on 52nd Street in NYC. I mainly rode on the New York subway back and forth from Manhattan to the New York airports to clear packages through customs. I can't remember why or how I got away with not going to work in the pretzel bakery that summer. Maybe the bakery business was gone by then, and my father was driving a taxi. I can't remember.

In the late spring of 1952 after I was graduated from high school, I finally escaped from summers with my parents by taking a job as a busboy and handyman at Seven Hills, a hotel in Lenox, Mass. I felt as if I had successfully run away from home, and I was delighted to be away.

Larry and Sophie Howitt were the owners of the place. I felt as if the Howitts, although they were tough bosses, had adopted me. They were not exactly my financial saviors early on. I was paid a mere pittance in salary, in addition to room and board, but I earned a little money in tips waiting on tables. The money I made was enough to pay the small portion of the Columbia College tuition that was not paid for by scholarships (my share of the total tuition was $400-600 then; yes, that's correct), and my living expenses while I lived at home during the school year.

At Seven Hills, besides waiting on tables I learned how to mow lawns, and to mingle with people with serious cultural interests, mainly New Yorkers coming to Seven Hills for its proximity to sites such as Tanglewood and Jacob's Pillow (dance festival). My interests were broadened by my fellow workers as well. Randy Weston, who doubled as a dishwasher, played piano at Seven Hills. He later became a famous jazz musician.

The sleeping quarters for help like me at Seven Hills were in a dirty disorganized barn down a short hill from the main house, in the woods. The ground was largely dirt and a few boards. At least here, I could sleep until seven AM instead of being awakened in the middle of the night like in my pretzel-bending days. Although there were a few unsettling occasions when a fellow employee, drunk and disorderly, shouted at the top of his lungs at the foot of my bed in the middle of the night.

The real saving grace of working at Seven Hills was being close to Tanglewood, the music festival, during the days of Lucas Foss and Leonard Bernstein. Being a teenager, lying on the cool grass on the outside lawn, listening to the Boston Symphony Orchestra and so many great soloists, under the stars. I was happy. Although I had no personal training in music, I have always loved classical music. My enjoyment of Tanglewood increased during subsequent summers at Seven Hills because of all I learned in and out of the core curriculum at Columbia College.

After several summers at Seven Hills, I tried working one summer as a waiter at a resort in the Catskill Mountains in New York State, again to earn the money I was responsible for in my tuition and to cover other expenses during the school year. I made good money, $2000-3000 in tips, but it was a frenetic work environment. I didn't like either the clientele or my fellow workers. The cut-throat competition among waiters in the Catskills, and the social shenanigans with guests at the hotels, often resulting in a lack of sleep and exhaustion, were not for me. It wasn't the same environment I had and appreciated at Seven Hills. I returned to Seven Hills during my last summers in medical school.

I needed no money from my parents. That I could pay my own tuition and expenses was a tremendously liberating situation. I feel very sad that college and medical students today cannot earn their way through school as I did. I think the sky-high costs and debt acquired during their education leave students today from the middle and lower middle classes like I was back then with an oppressively heavy burden as they enter their careers. I had no such burden and did not feel weighed down by continuing debt as they must feel.

However, since I needed to earn money, I never had the luxury of working in a laboratory or hospital or of taking courses during summers in medical school. I can still remember that during my first year at Harvard Medical School, I felt inferior in only one way to my fellow students: I had never taken advanced science courses in college or had any previous experience in medicine or science. I first learned my science and medicine in my classes in medical school, and sometimes from classmates like Jordie Cohen who taught me how to use the microscope. But my overall medical school record was good enough to earn me admission to Alpha Omega Alpha, a national medical honor society, so it all worked out fine in the end.

Love and marriage

I met my future wife during my second year in medical school. I thought she was beautiful, intelligent, independent-minded and sincere. In the first week of our relationship, I knew I wanted to be with her forever. We met in Cambridge while she was in a work program that was part of her college curriculum. When she left Cambridge, I spent as much time as I could driving in my battered old blue Oldsmobile back and forth between our schools. We were married the same week I was graduated.

Our personal life has been good to us. We have been married 52 years and have two grown sons, and three grandchildren. Thanks to my scientific career, we have been able to travel quite a bit, mainly because I was invited to lecture and participate in conferences around the world.

CHAPTER SIX

Basic Training

I applied to many hospitals for medical internship and residency training. My first four choices were Presbyterian Hospital and New York Hospital in New York, and Massachusetts General and the Peter Bent Brigham in Boston. The Harvard (II and IV) Medical Service at the Boston City Hospital (BCH) was next and that was the program highest on my list to which I was accepted. I have always felt lucky that I was chosen to be there.

Not only were we trained to treat patients with an extremely broad range of acute and chronic medical conditions, we saw these conditions in spades. Patients with infectious diseases: pneumonias, tuberculosis and fungal disorders. Also patients with diabetes and common cardiac conditions like heart attacks, hypertension and congestive heart failure. Of course, I also became an expert on alcoholism and its complications: delirium tremens (DTs), severe liver disease with bleeding varicose veins, and related mental disorders like Korsakoff's psychosis. The BCH provided the ultimate medical training experience. I was not surprised to read years later that this training program produced a great many professors of medicine.

I had never worked at the BCH during my medical school years. While during the last two years at Harvard Medical School I had many clinical experiences in medicine, nothing prepared me for the intensity of my internship and residency at the Boston City Hospital. Internship was like being simultaneously in boot camp in basic training and on active duty in a war zone. The days and nights consisted of constant activity, treating medical disaster after medical disaster.

I was busy taking care of very sick ward patients, almost full-time. When the phone rang on the ward, a disembodied voice said, "You have a DL on the accident floor." That was the shorthand for the fact that I had a new patient on the danger list (DL) whom I had to go down to the emergency room to see and escort to my ward and care for. There were no intensive care units (ICUs) back then. The medical wards were the ICUs. Similarly, there were no cardiac intensive care units (CCUs) back then either. We, the house staff then, were the first and only line of treatment for very sick medical patients. As an intern, I was the main doctor on the case. I was expected to do everything, from the patients' blood counts to taking them down to radiology for their x-rays. Not just metaphorically, the patient was in my hands.

The BCH had a house staff coverage system in which the work-up of admissions to the medical wards after a certain time (11 PM, I think) was the responsibility of a particular intern assigned to that job, the so-called night float. He (there were no female interns or residents that I recall at the BCH back then) also was responsible for all emergencies that occurred at night in the care of patients on the wards.

The night float had an assigned room in the hospital in which he could sleep if he wasn't busy, which wasn't very often. The night float's worst nightmare, certainly mine, was receiving the dreaded phone call that said "You have a DL on the accident floor..." It meant that for the next few hours I would essentially be on my own with a sick patient who was an emergency admission. It was never considered good form to wake the assistant resident, my superior, also on duty in the hospital, to help with the new case, unless things really got out of hand. He was usually either playing poker with other residents on duty from other services, or sleeping, but was not expected to be disturbed.

You could have a rare good night as a night float and get no admissions and no phone calls from nurses on the ward regarding changing specific orders on patients or calls to see patients who were deteriorating or calls reporting leaking IVs that needed to be re-inserted properly. But it would be rare. On the other hand, you could get two or three new admissions and/or several phone calls about patients already on the wards a night. Hearing the phone ring as a night float was not welcome. For many years after my internship, the sound of the telephone ringing unexpectedly in general, and especially late at night, froze me almost instantaneously.

Some residents assigned to the wards, who were in charge of accepting patients for admission, would try to manipulate the night float system to their advantage. If 11 PM was the cut-off time for ward admissions, they would try to influence the emergency room staff or even the elevator operators to see to it that the patient would arrive on the medical floor after 11 PM, so that the night float, not their own ward team, was responsible for the patient's work-up, and they were off the hook. Certain house officers were notorious for this activity, they were well-known and thoroughly disliked. But most of the time, there was easy collegiality and sharing of responsibility among the medical house staff.

I thought the night float system was a good idea. It spared the intern on call who had worked all day from working all night as well. And the night float job, per se, was a change for the intern from the pressures of caring for a ward full of patients, all day, every day. The night float would arrive just before his appointed starting time, and stay through morning ward rounds the next day when he would present the new cases and overnight problems to the ward service team taking over.

The only downside of the night float system was its effect on continuity of patient care, a critically important issue in the care of all patients, especially acutely ill patients. You, as the night float, had worked up the patient, knew the history, did the physical, ordered the lab tests, administered treatment all night; then suddenly, the next day you were gone and the patient's care was turned over to a doctor who had never seen the patient before and whom the patient did not know. That was a problem. Because of this situation, patients admitted via the night float sometimes received inferior initial care from the intern who inherited them: either because the patient was less well-known to the intern or because the intern felt a little less responsibility for the patient, having not admitted him or her.

Emergencies

There were very few elective admissions to the hospital at the BCH. They were mostly emergencies. The emergency room itself was a nightmare for doctors as well as patients. There was an almost constant flow of patients there, the BCH being the major public hospital in Boston. Many of the patients seen at the BCH ER all year round were alcoholics who were brought in by the police with either acute problems, or who were just being delivered to the hospital as vagrants to be cared for after being found on the streets.

There were also many patients with trauma, but I don't remember ever being responsible for them. Surgical emergencies were handled separately. As a medical intern in the ER I only remember dealing with medical patients. Patients with acute medical problems such as bacterial pneumonias with high fever, recent heart attacks in shock, or congestive heart failure were rapidly processed and sent up to the interns on the wards with the familiar phone call, "You have a DL on the accident floor." If an alcoholic were shaking with delirium tremens (DTs), shaking and/or delusional, he (I don't remember many female alcoholics) would be rapidly admitted as well.

While rotating through the ER, I, and my fellow house officers found that there were many alcoholics who appeared in the ER who were so inebriated that they were difficult to categorize and to accurately triage. We weren't sure how acutely ill they were. They didn't all need to be admitted. Most of them were placed in a special room unceremoniously known through the years as "the tank." There, alcoholics who were simply anaesthetized from their alcohol, deeply drunk, could sleep off their stupors and did.

The major problem with this system was that we sometimes did not know what was wrong with the alcoholics who we put in this room. Mostly, we were correct in our assumption that they were simply alcoholics needing to sleep off their stupor. But occasionally this assumption was seriously wrong. If it were an extra busy time in the ER, we could not check on these patients as much as we should have, and a few expired from an undiagnosed stroke, heart attack or other condition. This never happened on my watch, but it could have, given the sheer volume of ER patients each of us had in the ER and the time limitations inevitably involved.

Patients, patience

Treating BCH patients admitted to the medical wards was more controlled and manageable than it was in the ER, but some ward patients were quite ornery and difficult to care for. I recall early in the internship,

Carl Silverman, one of the gentlest interns of us all, was spit in the face by a double amputee, a diabetic patient he was trying to treat. Carl just wiped his face and cleaned his glasses and continued on with his work. That image is the worst I have carried with me from the BCH.

Another condition that went with the BCH territory was the recidivism in the alcoholic population. So many alcoholics who were cared for intensely both physically and emotionally by many of us seemed to be caught up in a revolving hospital door. We got to know them; talked to them; treated them kindly. When they were well, we discharged them to support programs including Alcoholics Anonymous, and they seemed to do well for months. Then, suddenly, they would reappear in the ER again, drunk again. It was frustrating to many of us, and disappointed us.

We became jaded and less emotionally responsive to them with time. We could only do so much. We could not repair their socioeconomic wounds or cure their dependency. This sense of helplessness often fuels the so-called GOMER (Get Out Of My Emergency Room) mentality in which house officers joke about medical situations among themselves. It was our response to the constant stress of acute pressured patient care. I make no excuses for it. It is wrong. But looking back, I understand that resorting to this kind of gallows humor away from patients was a safety valve for us, a way to retain our sanity and to bond with each other, establishing a camaraderie that fortified us individually.

One patient I clearly recall treating was a man I brought up to the ward, after receiving the dreaded phone call, "You have a DL on the accident floor," who was having uncontrollable seizures. When we had the patient in bed on the ward and he was still seizing, the resident supervising me told me to fill a syringe with phenobarbital and start pushing it intravenously. I was so panicked I listened. I pushed and pushed. Yes, the patient eventually did stop seizing; but he also stopped breathing. We quickly called anesthesiology and the patient was intubated and did well, but it provided an important lesson to me. Think about all the consequences before you act, even in a desperate situation. And don't necessarily listen to your "superior."

We performed mouth-to-mouth resuscitation on the patient while we waited the minutes it took for the anesthesiologist to arrive. These were the days before formal CPR. Very occasionally, as in this case, the resuscitation worked as a desperate emergency measure. Most often, it did not. Also, at the BCH in those days, this procedure carried the risk of exposing each of us to tuberculosis, a not uncommon ailment of BCH patients then. We all used to carefully review the lab slips containing the results of sputum samples we had sent on patients suspected of tuberculosis; some were occasionally positive. I don't recall any house staff member who acquired active tuberculosis that way when I was a BCH house officer, but who knows?

The staff

I thought the house staff with me on the II and IV Medical Services, the Harvard services at the BCH, was remarkable. There were two other medical services representing Tufts and Boston University medical schools working at the BCH and they were also very competent, but I mainly knew the Harvard Service. I still fondly remember most of my intern mates. Our superiors, the assistant residents and residents (one and two years ahead of us) on the house staff were a memorable group as well. I remember Matty Scharff best. He was very thoughtful and helpful to me as an intern and in thinking about my future career. He became a professor at Albert Einstein medical school. We remained friends for many years. I also recall Don Summers and Steve Robinson as residents whom I respected and who taught me a lot.

I was a smoker in those days and frequently had a cough. Once, I thought I had pneumonia, and I went to Steve, who was a senior resident, two years ahead of me, to get examined, and hopefully, sent home to rest. He said: "You have a few rhonchi (abnormal breath sounds), but no pneumonia. Get back to work." If he had let me off, some other intern would have had to do extra duty to fill in for me; there were no alternates on this jury. Steve, who was a great teacher and clinician at Harvard and at the Beth Israel Hospital in later years, told me something about myself when we were together at the BCH that always registered with me as being true. He said, "Whenever any little thing happens to you that's good, it's the greatest thing in the whole world and you talk about it forever. And whenever even the littlest bad thing happens to you, it's as if it's the worst thing in the world." I didn't mind my moody ups and downs, although I can't say the same for everyone else I lived with or worked with.

If the house staff at the BCH were as remarkable as I thought, then the medical leaders when I was there would have to be described as superb. I had many important role models at the BCH as both a physician and the future scientist I would become. William B. Castle, one of the most preeminent physicians and clinical scientists in the world, was head of the Harvard Medical Service when I was there, He had helped discover the cause of pernicious anemia, vitamin B12 deficiency, and he had helped Linus Pauling figure out what caused sickle cell anemia.

But I remember Dr. Castle best on the same lunch line at the BCH with the rest of us, the hospital staff, including the interns and residents. He was always saying, "Excuse me," as he stepped aside to have us younger men and women in white go through for lunch. He thought we were busier than he was and should go first. He was always so civilized and related to us as equals despite his prominence.

Once, I had to meet with Dr. Castle one on one. The meeting occurred after an altercation I had with a parking attendant. I drove right past the attendant into the BCH parking lot and parked my car despite his refusal to give me the OK to do so, on the erroneous grounds that there were no parking spaces left. I was immediately reported. I was scared, but Dr. Castle was as gentle and understanding as he could be. Essentially, he told me not to do it again, and that was that. He was always friendly, cordial, approachable, although I don't remember a specific medical or scientific conversation I ever had with him. What I learned most from Bill Castle was to respect the younger people that I worked with in medicine and science and I always did. I never played father superior; at least I hope not. But I did have a much worse temper than Bill Castle. I never saw him angry, while I certainly could be.

Rudi Schmid, one of my attendings at the BCH, was my ideal role model as a scientist and clinician. He was always smiling, friendly, enthusiastic, and incredibly knowledgeable about everything; like Dr. Castle and most of the BCH faculty, he was easily approachable. He was an internationally-known scientist and yet he was very down-to-earth. Among his many research accomplishments, he had discovered an important liver enzyme necessary for bilirubin metabolism. He was a fine clinician as well. He was a really handsome man with a wonderful sense of humor.

I remember one day Dr. Schmid told us residents about a job offer he had received to be head of medicine at a very prestigious institution in his native Switzerland. The position was both a scientific and clinical professorship, and he went there for a visit. He said: "They wheeled a patient into rounds in an amphitheater. I was seated in the front row and after presentation of the patient, I alone was asked to make comments about diagnosis, treatment, background — anything I wanted. Then the patient was wheeled out. No discussion. No questions. I could never take a job in an atmosphere like that." He loved the give and take of American medicine and science, especially of the quality at the BCH and Harvard Medical School.

Rudi always had a smile, an insight, a great judgment, and he looked like he was having fun with everything. That was the most important thing I learned from him. You have to have fun with what you're doing professionally, even if it's a hard or stressful job. He later became dean of the medical school at UCSF and a major figure in liver transplantation.

Charley Davidson and Max Finland were two of my other favorite faculty members at BCH. Max was short and round; Charley tall and thin. They were nicknamed Mutt and Jeff. They were very different yet equally impressive and dynamic as physicians. Charley was an outstanding liver specialist. Charley's "Ho,ho,ho" chuckle and big open smile to almost everything could be punctuated suddenly with a serious and bitingly wry comment. He was head of one of the two Harvard medical services (the one I was in, the II Medical Service). He was always in charge, and accessible and smart.

Max, a world-famous genius in infectious diseases, was another great attending physician as well as scientist. I remember the first time I had a patient suspected of having subacute bacterial endocarditis, a serious blood infection, and he was the attending physician. He said, "Do six blood cultures," when asked how many blood samples to draw. "Why?" he was asked. "Because that's the right number. It ensures you get it right," he said, and he would quote the scientific literature chapter and verse to support his reasoning. "Sometimes, the result will be that six out of six cultures are positive, that's fine; but if it is only one positive out of six, you have to suspect contamination of the sample." He almost never smiled, but he did have a sense of humor. He would be unhappy, however, if you didn't do exactly what he said to do for a patient. He would always check with you the next day about the result. I learned an incredible amount about infectious diseases, especially about pneumococcal pneumonia and tuberculosis from Max Finland.

There were many more physicians who did teaching, medicine and science that I learned from at BCH. My first exposure to a super hematologist was when I was taught by Jim Jandl. I also managed to learn about renal disease while at the BCH from Arnold Relman who knew everything about the kidney. He was at Boston University School of Medicine then, but still listened to our problem cases. He subsequently became editor of the New England Journal of Medicine and a professor at Harvard Medical School, and he has written extensively about the ethical, economic, and social aspects of health care. He has been a strong advocate for limiting the influence of commercialism and for-profit entities in medicine, and to this day I have always been in synch with his views.

Most of the BCH attendings were incredibly diligent about supporting the house staff medically and emotionally. They were interested in patient care and education, and were usually researchers as well. They were my heroes, the so-called triple threats that I tried to emulate in my own career.

When I was done with my two years at the Boston City Hospital I was ready for anything in medicine. My two years there had prepared me for any medical emergencies I might confront in the future, and the proper ways to confront them. The two years I then spent at the National Institutes of Health (NIH) doing medical research were both a much needed break for me from the war zone of acute medical practice and the gateway to my career as a scientist as well as a physician in hematology and academic medicine in the following 40 plus years at Columbia Presbyterian.

PART THREE

Doing Medicine

CHAPTER SEVEN

A Special Calling

The practice of medicine is a special calling: like that of a priest, rabbi or teacher. In theory, medicine is the most selfless and self-fulfilling profession. It is the only profession in which the sole goal in its purest sense is to help the patient, and ideally there are no limits to the objectivity of the practitioner in focusing solely on that single-minded goal. There is a right answer to almost every patient's problem. And the only goal of the physician, again in theory, is to find that answer, the cause of the illness, and to cure that illness; and if there is no cure, to manage the illness in the best way possible. Find the cause, execute the proper orders, medicines, operations, etc., and restore, to the greatest extent possible, the patient's health. These aspirations are at the heart of always keeping the best interests of the patient in mind. No other considerations should enter the process or the decisions.

Medicine in theory is such a satisfying pursuit, both professionally and personally, that I think it should be considered by most of us as a calling if we are interested in and capable of practicing it. It is doing the most fruitful and fulfilling acts of all for our fellow men and women that I am aware of; it taps into all of one's talents, intelligence, skill, energy and emotional resources to treat and cure a fellow human being of his or her ailments. The practice of medicine offers a most gratifying life. While it requires a long period of training and preparation, it also provides economic stability for its practitioners. I have always been proud to be a physician.

As human beings, we all deserve the best medical care when we are sick. In the best of health care systems, we would all receive comfort as well as care as an integral part of treatment for our illnesses; no matter who we are. No one is immune to the need for comfort and care when they are sick. Everyone of us eventually has a fatal disease. That is the human condition. As human beings, we will be sick and we deserve to be comforted and cared for when we are sick. We need the best doctors to take care of us and to allay our anxieties when we are patients.

As patients, we all want the best medical care available to us. What is required for that care? The most important element is that each of us has the security that he or she will receive excellent and prompt medical care at any time it is needed. Optimal medical care is a right, not a privilege. The first and most important part of that care is that each of us has an empathetic and competent physician, an internist or pediatrician or general medical doctor available to us on demand. The second is that the institution at which we receive medical care is of high quality.

The Ideal Physician

What are the skills necessary?
What is the intelligence needed?
What is the emotional state required?

I have very high standards for the ideal physician, and I certainly don't meet them all. But they are what I hope my own physicians and surgeons come closest to meeting, if at all possible. The ideal physician must be as empathetic as a most trusted confidant and as intelligent and probing as a scientist. The patient should be the doctor's only concern, and helping the patient the only goal. To do this, the doctor must be entirely focused on the patient and his or her problems — psychological, physical, emotional. The doctor has to make the patient feel comfortable enough to tell his or her story in its entirety. The doctor must never be too busy or rushed, except in rare emergencies, to listen to the patient's concerns intently and completely. The doctor must leave his ego outside the room.

If the patient doesn't think the doctor cares much about him or her as a patient, there can be no meaningful doctor-patient relationship. The patient must trust that the doctor is really listening. The doctor has to convey the feeling that he or she is completely focused on what the patient is saying with all of his or her whole mind while at the same time processing the patient's complaints and symptoms.

The ideal physician must also be concentrating solely on the patient when he or she does the physical exam. As I was told early in my training, "If you don't look under the patient's tongue and ask yourself, 'Is there anything under the patient's tongue,' you're not going to miraculously see what's under the patient's tongue.'" You have to look in order to see.

So, in the doctor-patient relationship, first, there must be empathy and trust; second, there must be concentration and focus on the patient's history and physical exam: the symptoms and signs.

But one also needs something more to be the ideal physician: one also needs intelligence and wisdom. Intelligence in figuring out what the patient has; wisdom in knowing how to communicate that knowledge to the patient. Both are necessary in knowing how to treat the malady.

Wisdom is a combination of knowledge and human feeling — both — not one without the other. It is true, as has been said many times, that medicine is both an art and a science. The physician must combine knowledge with empathy and concern, individualized to the patient's needs, giving no less care to the patient than the physician would want if the patient were his or her own self or a family member or loved one.

The good physician never leaves decisions about care of the patient to the patient or family alone. If there are different choices that can be made in a patient's care, the good doctor presents them, but always finishes his or her discussion with the patient and/or the family with his or her own point of view. The end of the discussion should include a line from the doctor like " I think it would be best if we did...(thus and so)." After all, the doctor is the expert, not the patient. The onus of decision-making should always be on the doctor, and in the best doctor-patient relationships this process relieves the patient and family of any personal feelings of blame or responsibility for the medical outcome.

The Drill: Taking the history

There is a well-established "drill," as I call it, to the evaluation of a medical patient, especially the first time a patient is seen during a hospital admission or in a first office visit. This drill or "work-up" is widely taught to medical students and widely used by house staff, and is supposedly ingrained in all of us as future physicians for the rest of our professional lives. It provides a standardized way to evaluate patients. The work-up includes the patient's medical history; the physical examination; standard laboratory tests; a list of possible diagnoses (the "differential diagnosis"); and a summary appraisal of the patient. This somewhat formalized process, in at least the initial evaluation of medical patients, should be used routinely by all physicians, but often is not. If it were, it would greatly improve the overall quality of medicine practiced by physicians.

The "Medical History," usually provided in a form for most physicians, usually starts with a "Chief Complaint (CC)" and a "Present Illness (PI)." The CC, "back pain," "vomiting," "a rash," is the main symptom or sign that brought the patient to the hospital or doctor's office. A symptom is subjective: something the patient feels; a sign is objective: something the patient sees or can be seen. Back pain or headaches are symptoms; rashes or lumps are signs. Most symptoms are elicited by the history; most signs on physical examination.

The CC is something the doctor must provide an explanation for in his or her final evaluation. It is the first step in taking the medical history. The next step is finding out everything about the present illness: when it started; does the CC and other symptoms and signs persist or wax and wane; how severe are they; are they associated with other symptoms and/ or signs? When? How?

Included in the PI, at least by me, is all the information about any other symptoms and signs related to the CC. If the CC is "vomiting," then the history of the PI should include related issues such as changes in bowel habits, the presence or absence of diarrhea, abdominal pain, etc. And the "etc" is a long established list of additional questions to be asked to further define the PI. All the relevant questions have to be asked by the physician in the area of the CC and PI, especially when a new patient is first seen for a significant new illness. The doctor must ask the patient these questions. Patients cannot and should not be expected to provide all of this information spontaneously. They also cannot be expected to know the meaning of the presence or absence of specific symptoms and signs in their illnesses. Patients are not doctors.

Many of the specific questions in the history are used to reveal so-called "pertinent negatives:" symptoms and signs that the patient doesn't have and which make certain diagnoses less likely; by the same token, those symptoms and signs, if present and positive, would make certain diagnoses more likely.

The patient may often not realize the significance or interconnection of symptoms and signs elicited by the physician's questions. If you don't ask a specific question as the physician, you may overlook significant history. You're the doctor. It's your job to obtain the full history; it's not the patient's job to spontaneously provide it. I don't think the average patient today is any smarter about their medical illness than they used to be. Nor should they be assumed to be, an assumption made by many physicians today, for reasons unknown to me, but perhaps erroneously related to the readily accessible medical information available on the Internet.

A complete history by itself will often lead the physician to a correct diagnosis. The process of taking a medical history is akin to being a detective. You have to elicit all of the facts without endangering the trust and cooperation of the patient. You must also get the whole true story as objectively as the patient knows it, including all of its potentially embarrassing details, if they exist. The patient must tell you the whole truth.

The history of the present illness entails reviewing many of the details of the patient's earlier medical history and life. As you hear the patients' stories, you must be probing in your questioning in order to elicit as many details as you can; you ask every question you think is necessary to define as precisely as possible past and present problems. By the time the PI is done, you should know what to look for in your physical examination and what lab tests you need to have done in order to arrive at a firm specific diagnosis. You need time and patience to do this; otherwise you may fail. This is a drill you have to get done right if you are to be successful in medical diagnosis.

The main problem in medical diagnosis today is that most physicians don't take the time or feel they have the time to obtain a complete medical history, and jump to conclusions too quickly. By not making detailed history-taking a routine part of their patient work-ups, physicians fall into bad habits. Many physicians rely on the responses of the patients to written questionnaires for most of their history-taking. The introduction of computerized history-taking is equally potentially dangerous to me. While these questionnaires can be initial guides, they seldom pick up the important details and nuances of the history that can lead to a diagnosis, especially in difficult cases. When responses are elicited directly by the doctor face-to-face with the patient, each response leads to another question in a much more logical manner. Without the benefit of a complete history, physicians today often rely on complicated tests like MRIs and CAT scans and even laparoscopies in seeking to replace the history and physical examination as a means to establish diagnoses. These tests are most useful to confirm and document diagnoses, but not in leading the physician to the logical answers to the patient's problems. These tests are unnecessary to establish most diagnoses.

In the first visit with a patient in the office or the hospital, the physician needs to follow the CC and PI by a "Review of Systems (ROS)," another attempt at completeness of history-taking. Questions are asked about other systems seemingly unrelated to the patient's present illness. However, this history may reveal unsuspected facts relevant to the PI for both doctor and patient. A previously unrevealed episode of illness may be uncovered during the review of systems that indeed is a clue to the present illness. For example, a forgotten fracture of the pelvis in the past may be relevant to the patient's current problems in the blood vessels of his leg.

The medical history also includes a "Social History," to elicit facts about smoking, drinking, marital status, travel, medications. These facts may also contain unsuspected clues. For example, in the course of the inquiry into the social history, exposure to infectious agents or poisons may be revealed. Also included in the History is a "Family History" to probe for information about possible genetic origins of disease. Again, while questionnaires can be guides to the ROS and Social History, the physician's direct questioning of the patient about pertinent positives and negatives is indispensible if the physician is to have all of the information necessary to insure the proper care of the patient.

Many times today, especially in academic medical settings, I have seen physicians accompanied by a medical student or another visitor, even when the doctor is seeing a patient for the first time. As an academic, I understand the need for this kind of mentorship by senior physicians of younger ones. However, as a patient, I always want my physician with me alone in the room. He or she is the one I trust with my care and to whom I can freely give all of the information about my illness without feeling embarrassed or exposed. I personally do not feel comfortable, in the office or the hospital as a patient, when people other than my doctor are present when I am seen. For me, medical care is personal, between my doctor and me.

The physical examination: a lost art

The physical examination is another critical part of the initial evaluation of the patient and often confirms the diagnostic clues provided by the medical history. In the same way that history-taking is carefully taught in most medical schools and training programs, so too is the performance of a proper physical examination. The fact is, again, some practicing physicians don't feel they have the time or need to do proper physical examinations. I was really shocked when one of my primary physicians during my illness never did a physical examination, even though he was an excellent physician in other areas of my care.

The physical examination is still a vital part of every patient's initial work-up and follow-up. This continues to be true even with the advent of more advanced medical imaging procedures in recent years that can reveal lesions (masses, defects) that, indeed, cannot be felt by physical examination. The idea that we should just throw people into sophisticated CAT scans or MRIs most of the time to make diagnoses or follow disease is just unnecessary and wrong. The expense of these procedures is not the only major issue. It is that they are often unnecessary for diagnosis or treatment; they can be harmful in exposure to radiation; and, if negative, can be falsely reassuring. They are often used by physicians to substitute for what they should be doing: taking the brief time needed to do an appropriate physical examination.

The physical examination (PE) usually starts from the head down in a predictable way. Obviously, if a patient is bleeding and in pain from a gash in his leg, I would start the physical there. However, despite the fact that the source of the patient's chief complaint may be the belly or the leg, my physical examination usually starts with evaluation of the skin and head and neck and moves south. Examination of the skin is first for me. Looking for rashes, bruises, lesions. The head exam includes looking at and in the eyes, nose, ears, mouth.

As with history-taking, physicians must be proactive in doing the physical examination. There are no labels on diseased or involved organs. As I've said before, if you want to see what is under the tongue, you have to concentrate for a second and look under the tongue. If you want to see what's in the retina of the eye, you need to use your ophthalmoscope and look there, specifically at the blood vessels there and at the margins of the optic disk. If you want to know whether the pupils react to light properly, you have to test them and be alert to the results.

Physicians are not usually endowed with any special powers of observation; they have to choose to use their learned skills; they have been trained to know what questions to ask and what to look for and they must put their training to proper use with every patient they see. There are no short cuts. Again, compulsivity and attention to detail are major assets.

There are, of course, some physicians who are more skilled at physical examination than others. I am not one of the very best. Physicians I have worked with have had more skill at certain aspects of physical examination than I have. Some physicians can hear more heart murmurs than I can, even when I am using their stethoscopes. This may be related to a hearing defect I have had for a number of years. But at least I have always tried to hear them, and I did hear most that were significant.

Some of my colleagues have felt more masses or seen more subtle skin lesions on PE than I. However, these and other often subtle defects in my skills do not justify my not doing the best physical exam I can in my evaluation of patients. I actually became more expert than most at detecting spleen tips on PE as a result of my long experience as a hematologist. If the spleen is felt on physical examination, under the rib cage on the left side with the patient taking a deep breath, then it is pathologically enlarged, and some medical explanation must be sought. The spleen is increased in size in certain blood disorders, like anemias or leukemias.

There is no rationale in my mind for the argument that doing a physical is a waste of time since imaging studies can reveal the same findings in greater detail. This argument is, rather, an excuse for the reduction in time and effort the physician wants to spend examining the patient. Also, even in this age of multi-tasking, there is a price for doing two things at the same time. I have to concentrate when I am doing a proper physical exam.

It is hard for me to do so if I am busy chatting with my patient about the latest film or sports event during the exam.

The physical exam done properly often reveals important clues to a diagnosis, if you look for them. In the mouth, you can see lesions; in the eyes, jaundice, pupil disorders, cataracts; on retinal examination, vascular diseases or bleeding; in the ears, wax. In the neck examination, masses, venous distention, artery integrity, the thyroid. In the chest, strange sounds called "rhonchi" and "rales" that indicate disease. Proper chest examination can reveal dullness that indicates the potential presence of pneumonia.

Sure, you're going to get a chest x-ray anyway if a patient comes in with a cough and fever and has findings on physical exam of the chest consistent with a diagnosis of pneumonia, but you will at least have some confirmation of pneumonia and the baseline physical findings that will allow you to re-evaluate the patient without having him or her get another chest x-ray every time you see the patient subsequently.

The same principles apply to the abdomen and the rest of the body. The physical examination can lead you towards a specific diagnosis. If you can localize the source of the patient's abdominal pain during a careful physical examination, that can be very important in the further work-up. If physical signs like tenderness during your examination point to the upper abdomen, then an ulcer or gall bladder disease are most likely. If the symptoms and signs are in the right lower quadrant, appendicitis is a leading possibility. If you feel any masses or organs, these are very helpful in pinpointing the source of the problem. For example, if the liver or spleen is felt on the PE, the enlargement of these organs is abnormal, and must be explained.

Feeling for hernias and a proper rectal examination in males is required on the first full visit or hospitalization as part of the PE. In females, pelvic and rectal examinations are most often done today by an obstetrician-gynecologist. In my early days as an internist, it was not uncommon for internists to do these examinations on the initial patient visit, with a nurse present, especially if other symptoms or signs pointed to possible disease in the involved areas.

A properly done PE helps to confirm or reject your diagnostic thinking that resulted from your evaluation of the patient's symptoms and signs by history. It can reveal objective signs that can confirm your diagnostic thinking. It also gives you a measure of the severity of the illness. If the doctor, for reasons of time or temperament, doesn't examine the patient, then he or she is ignoring potentially vital information that can help arrive at a correct diagnosis.

I was always a very busy physician when I was caring for patients as an attending physician, because of my other responsibilities as a scientist and director of a big research laboratory, and of a division in the department of medicine and as a laboratory administrator, but I seldom left a new patient's bedside for the first time as a ward attending without performing a physical examination that at least included the area the patient complained about, and the chest and abdomen; and when I couldn't do it right there and then, I promised to come back and do so soon, and I did.

The laboratory and x-rays: great advances

After taking a history and doing a physical examination, laboratory tests and x-rays are used to confirm or pinpoint diagnoses. There have been enormous advances in diagnostic testing over the past half century. These, together with so many new effective treatments, have led to great advances in the practice of medicine. However, these advances do not, as many physicians now think, make compulsive and accurate history-taking and physical examination of the patient, any less important. These old-fashioned aspects of medicine point the way to the pertinent laboratory tests that should be done. Newer more advanced radiologic tests, the CAT scan, or the MRI, may, in turn, pinpoint and establish the diagnosis precisely and quickly, and lead to the prompt institution of proper treatment.

However, a shotgun approach to using advanced medical imaging techniques like total body scanning or multiple unnecessary laboratory tests and diagnostic procedures is no substitute for the physician obtaining a proper history and doing a proper physical examination. This is true, not only because this approach increases the cost of medical care enormously, but, more importantly, because it often is ineffective and inefficient medical practice leading to mindless medicine.

In addition, high-tech approaches often lead to medical mistakes with many false positive results leading to new blind alleys and unnecessary treatments, which are not risk-free. Doctors who practice in this way should be held accountable for these mistakes.

Laboratory tests and radiologic (x-ray) studies are most often necessary to make or confirm most diagnoses. They often provide the "pathognomonic" feature, the feature absolutely characteristic of the disease, required to make a firm diagnosis. The patient may give a good history of cough and fever, and you may hear rales or rhonchi or the lack of breath sounds on physical examination of the chest. But it is the chest x-ray and sputum culture that will confirm the diagnosis of pneumonia; the latter, if positive, will identify the offending bacteria. And the x-ray, if positive, will reveal the pneumonia. They are the critical features that make the diagnosis certain.

It is also true that you do not have to wait for the sputum or blood culture results to be available before you treat the patient, although you should do all of the necessary bacteriological testing before starting antibiotics. If you do not do the bacterial cultures before you start treatment, cultures done while a patient is on antibiotics may not reveal the offending organism because the antibiotics given to the patient can suppress the growth of the organism in the culture. The prescribed antibiotics may not, at the same time, cure the infection in the patient. When this happens, it is necessary to stop the ineffective antibiotics, repeat the bacterial cultures, and then start new antibiotic treatment.

Characteristic changes on an electrocardiogram (ECG, EKG) are pathognomonic for the diagnosis of a heart attack. Other findings such as enzyme changes on laboratory tests may confirm the diagnosis, but the ECG establishes it. You may need further evaluation of the coronary arteries with angiography and other testing for more precisely defining the heart damage, but the ECG establishes the diagnosis.

Diagnosing masses (lumps or tumors), seen or felt raise other diagnostic issues. A biopsy with typical pathological findings makes the diagnosis of most tumors. Masses can be caused by a vast array of benign (non-malignant) conditions including acute and chronic infections, and some tumors can masquerade as others. If, for instance, you think the patient's lumps are due to lymph node enlargement caused by infectious mononucleosis and you have other clinical and laboratory evidence for that diagnosis, you don't need to perform a lymph node biopsy. However, when a mass is not the result of an obvious infectious or inflammatory process and persists and malignancy is suspected, it is absolutely critical that a biopsy be done for diagnosis. Nothing less is adequate. Every diagnosis of every malignant tumor must be confirmed by biopsy before definitive anti-tumor treatment is begun. If you're going to give a patient radiation therapy or chemotherapy, you need a biopsy and a pathological diagnosis before doing so.

It isn't necessary to have an absolutely secure diagnosis when treating a patient for relatively minor illnesses. Doctors see many patients in their offices for a variety of symptoms and diseases like viral illnesses, muscle strains, headaches and the like and treat them symptomatically. If symptoms improve, fine. If not, the patient needs a more thorough evaluation.

I am not trying to be exhaustive in expressing my thoughts on the practice of general internal medicine. I am just trying to indicate the approach that I used as a practitioner, which I think is still useful to know about today.

The science of medicine

Internal medicine is incredibly complicated on the one hand, and yet not incomprehensibly so, on the other. There are only a finite number of possibilities in medical diagnosis. If you acquire all the facts you need to know; if you're focused on the goal of arriving at a correct diagnosis; and if you think logically every step of the way, you'll do fine.

In this respect, the practice of medicine is a science. Medical diagnosis shares many features with laboratory science. I have been absorbed intellectually and emotionally in both fields, and feel that they have common threads. You have to be well trained and knowledgeable in both areas, and both areas require a systematic approach. Devising experiments to answer a specific biological question requires the same rigorous mental processing that must be followed when seeing patients and arriving at the medical diagnosis. In science, you devise the experiment carefully and with controls, making sure you can conclude something from it, no matter the result. In medicine, you take the history, do the physical exam, do tests and also must come to a conclusion.

In both science and medicine, you use all of your previous fund of information; concentrate; obsess; leave little to chance, make sure you ask all the right questions; come to logical conclusions in examining the results. I have always thought that my experiences and expertise in clinical medicine and those in laboratory research complemented each other. In all of my clinical activities as an academic physician caring for patients, I always had an open dialogue with other physicians, students, house staff and fellows in much the same way I did with my colleagues in my laboratory life. I always welcomed the contributions and opinions of others. In both settings, however, when I was in charge, I was often the most vocal in expressing my own opinions and, of course, in deciding how to either treat the patient, or do and interpret an experiment. While I always listened to and respected others' points of view, I always said my piece and held my ground when I thought that I was right. I would have made a terrible politician, and seldom tried to be one, in either my medical or scientific endeavors.

A major difference between being a clinician and being a scientist is that time is of the essence in medical diagnosis and treatment while it is much less so in research. In addition, in medicine, doctors are often helped by their patients since patients often get better by themselves. By contrast, in the laboratory, no such help is provided; no results are obtained spontaneously or very quickly. It often took me years to answer basic questions about the pathophysiology of disorders of human hemoglobin I had under study in the laboratory. One doesn't have that kind of time to make a proper useful diagnosis with patients and to treat them. You have to be quick and accurate. I sometimes had instant satisfaction from successfully diagnosing and treating patients. Satisfaction in the laboratory, by contrast, usually came only after months and even years of work. I never was sure if or when or from where my satisfaction would come. On the lighter side, like many of my colleagues who did both clinical medicine and laboratory research, I was the subject of an old joke: I was a great clinician to my scientific colleagues, and a great scientist to my clinical associates.

CHAPTER EIGHT

Making Diagnoses

There are only so many organ systems in our bodies for physicians to worry about: dermatologic (skin); cardiac (heart); pulmonary (lungs); gastro-intestinal (GI, digestive); orthopedic (bones and joints); rheumatic (inflammatory and immunologic); vascular (blood vessels); infectious; neurologic (brain and nerves); psychiatric (mental function); hematologic (blood system); oncologic (cancer, not really a system but a specialty); genitourinary; gynecologic (women's organs). The good diagnostician has information about all of these systems as known chapters etched in his or her mind, available to be accessed instantaneously on seeing a new patient with a new problem.

Most patients have a discrete chief complaint suggesting involvement of one or a few particular organ systems: "I have chest pain," tells the doctor that the patient has a problem with either the heart, lungs or nervous system. "I have pain in my belly" tells the doctor that the patient has problems with digestive, urinary or genital systems. While asking the questions the doctor is going through his mental computer narrowing the possibilities that explain the particular array of symptoms. Having done this so many times during training, the good physician homes in on the correct diagnosis fairly quickly...but never too quickly.

As in any other logical process, good physicians build their case for a logical diagnosis by adding individual pieces of evidence to bolster their case, and eventually obtain enough evidence to either prove it or to reject it. The physician must have an absolutely open mind until he or she has the diagnosis.

In most cases, making a diagnosis is relatively easy. If the patient presents with chest pain, shortness of breath and fever, you focus on the cardio-respiratory system in your thinking. Is it a heart attack? Pneumonia?

A pulmonary embolus (blockage of blood vessels with blood clots)? You ask all the questions about the patient's possible lung or heart problems; you go through the drill. Then you do a physical examination to try to see if there is physical evidence to support your hunches. You examine the chest, and listen for abnormal sounds that are common with pneumonia. But those sounds may also occur with heart failure consistent with a heart attack.

You listen for weak or irregular heart sounds which might support the diagnosis of a heart attack. Then you do a chest x-ray and an electrocardiogram (ECG) and specific laboratory tests to try to arrive at a firm specific diagnosis. If the chest x-ray shows certain shadows associated with pneumonia, you may have made a diagnosis. A positive sputum culture showing pneumonia-causing bacteria will confirm the diagnosis and define the specific type of pneumonia.

On the other hand, the chest x-ray may show no pneumonia, but other changes in the lungs consistent with a heart attack. If the ECG shows certain pathologic changes, you may have the cardinal features of a heart attack. Special blood tests will confirm the diagnosis.

As I said earlier, the positive chest x-ray and bacterial cultures on the one hand, and diagnostic ECG changes on the other in other, are pathognomonic: they are specific findings that make the diagnosis certain. You have confirmed your suspicions: you have a diagnosis and are ready to treat the patient. Patients with heart attacks must be hospitalized. If the patient has a treatable pneumonia, you may or may not hospitalize the patient.

If the chest x-ray and ECG are normal or non-diagnostic in the patient with chest pain, shortness of breath and fever, at least you have ruled out the most common treatable and serious diagnoses. But now, you must continue to search for a cause of the chest pain and shortness of breath. You must quickly rule out a pulmonary embolus (a clot in the lungs) using special diagnostic tests that include further x-ray studies. Pulmonary emboli, if present, will require immediate treatment with anticoagulation (blood thinners) or even surgery to avoid potential medical catastrophe.

If you still don't have an answer after all of your testing, then you observe the patient closely in the hospital if they are seriously ill. You will watch to see what happens, and, perhaps, think of other diagnoses, such as viral disease, or vascular problems. If the symptoms and signs fade, you might call the whole episode viral or just settle for the diagnosis of an unexplained illness. But if the patient's symptoms and signs persist, you may have to dig deeper for a correct diagnosis: has the patient been exposed to rare pathogens (infectious agents) or toxins (poisons)? Is it lung cancer or tuberculosis, the great masquerader? Where has the patient been and who and what have they been exposed to? Do you consider a biopsy of the heart or lung? The search goes on. Sometimes no answer is found. But no answer should be the last thing on your mind as the physician, especially if the illness does not improve with treatment.

In a different scenario, if the patient enters with nausea, vomiting, and/ or abdominal pain, you are focused on the gastrointestinal (GI) system. Again, you use the medical history to find out in detail when the symptoms occur; where the pain is located; how long has the illness been present. Then you try to confirm the origin of the pain by examining the abdomen carefully. If pain and tenderness are located in the right upper quadrant, then the problem is likely to be gall bladder disease or a liver problem. If on the left, the gall bladder is less likely to be the cause.

If symptoms and signs are below the chest in the midline, it's more likely to be the stomach or upper intestine (duodenum). Maybe an ulcer, gastritis, or a viral illness. Again, you use x-rays and blood and other laboratory tests to try to establish and/or confirm your diagnosis. If there is clearly an ulcer seen on x-ray (upper GI series) and/or gastroscopy (looking at the GI tract via a tube), then you have a diagnosis. If, on the other hand, there are gallstones present, they will usually be seen by x-ray; gall bladder disease is the likely culprit for the symptoms and signs. Again, if a firm diagnosis is not established, you think more; get more history if you can; do more tests.

These are examples of relatively simple type cases that constitute the vast majority of common medical illnesses. The organ system involved is clear. In most cases, the history is the single most important initial source of information and will direct the doctor to do a physical examination and then appropriate tests to determine the source of the medical problem and to arrive at a correct diagnosis.

Good judgment is the final necessary ingredient in the process. Sadly, while most doctors will go through the diagnostic process and come to the correct diagnosis, some lack good judgment and come to erroneous diagnoses.

The Difficult Cases

The physician's best friend is the ability of the human body to heal itself: to successfully overcome disease spontaneously, without treatment. Many of our minor ailments are cured by the body's natural defenses, especially the work of the immune system and our normal blood cells. These illnesses include viral infections, and pathologic processes like inflammation or trauma which often respond to watchful waiting, and/or to pain medication and anti-inflammatory drugs.

However, there are also many cases in medicine in which the disease does not go away, and in which the diagnosis is not obvious. These difficult cases are the most challenging for internists and medical specialists like me. They really are detective stories. Most of them can be satisfactorily solved, and the patients appropriately treated. As I have said, there are only so many organ systems for diagnosticians to worry about: cardio-respiratory; gastrointestinal; infectious; genitourinary; neurologic; hematologic; musculoskeletal; immunologic; endocrine; psychiatric. And there are specialists, experts in each of these areas, who are especially trained and experienced to solve particular cases.

Many of these cases involve more than one system; they are so-called "multisystem" or "systemic" diseases, and some of these are of unknown origin. Almost every type of case under the sun has been reported somewhere in the medical literature, and, indeed, most complex cases can be treated successfully after diagnosis by the expert physician.

Again, the physician only discovers what he or she looks for. There is no substitute for experience in many of these cases. If you've seen a rare disease as the diagnosis in one or two previous cases, your brain is more likely to put together the information that suggests to you that this same diagnosis may be present in a currently puzzling unsolved case. Going to computer-based diagnostics may be helpful to the medical expert occasionally to review the possible causes for a symptom complex, but using the detailed history and physical examination and your memory will probably be more productive.

Most of these cases of systemic or multisystem disease are spread through the body by the blood stream or lymph nodes. They manifest themselves in many organ systems. For example, tuberculosis is an infectious disease that starts in the lungs, but can disseminate; it can invade the lymph glands; it can spread through the blood to the bone marrow, and can be present in almost any other organ as well. Its presence as the cause of disease in these organs is unusual and, thus, difficult to diagnose. Tuberculosis is, therefore, known in diagnostic medical lingo as "the great masquerader" because it can mimic so many other illnesses.

While I was a house officer at the BCH, I had a few cases of disseminated tuberculosis with unusual presentations, once with masses (lymph nodes) eroding into the chest wall. The diagnosis seemed to be cancer, but a biopsy of the mass revealed tuberculosis. I was so struck by this and other cases of disseminated tuberculosis I had seen that when I came to PH and a patient came in with a complicated illness, constituting a difficult multisystem case, I would almost always suggest ruling out tuberculosis. The fact is, I never saw a case of disseminated tuberculosis in all of my time at PH. I sometimes noted smirks from my colleagues when I suggested the diagnosis once too often in difficult unsolved cases, but I'm still glad I thought of it when I did. It is a treatable and potentially curable disease, even when disseminated, but only when the diagnosis is made.

Other multisystem diseases include other infectious diseases. I made the diagnosis of leprosy on the medical wards of PH once, a rarity in the US. Other multisystem diseases can be immunologically-based diseases of lymphocytes: antibody producing B cells or tissue T lymphocytes; diseases of blood vessels and related tissues (vasculitis), some of which may also be caused by immune dysfunction; malignancies including leukemias, lymphomas and metastatic solid tumors (lung, breast, colon, etc.); and many rarer conditions.

In some complex cases, the history may point to one or more systems but the medical evaluation doesn't confirm a simple diagnosis. The patient with nausea, vomiting and abdominal pain doesn't turn out to have an ulcer or gall bladder disease or a viral illness. What then? Well then you have to probe more intensely into the history and find out what really is going on.

And you have to start thinking about those rarer conditions that might be present. An old expression in medicine is: "When you hear hoof beats, don't think of zebras!" That is, when a diagnosis is sought, you usually think of the more common conditions. But when none of the common diagnoses for the patient's symptoms fit, then you must think of the unusual.

In my experience, the answer often can be found in exploring the history more deeply. Not just asking when did the illness start, but under what precise conditions? Was it related to any particular conditions that the patient was exposed to at the time? Eating certain foods? Taking certain medicines? Traveling somewhere unusual? Changing certain habits? Using new detergents? Having contacts, sexual or other, temporally related to the onset of the illness? Was the patient exposed to a rare virus or bacteria or other toxic substance? Does he or she have acute intermittent porphyria, a rare diagnosis associated with episodes of nausea and vomiting? Or does he or she have another one of the other many rare diseases?

My approach in these cases is to think about the "pathophysiology" of the illness and then translate that into a diagnosis. The pathophysiology is the biological process that leads to the pathology of the disease. I try to find out what started the pathologic process and then figure out how that inciting event led to the development of other changes which are reflected in the patient's symptoms and signs.

In a patient with a heart attack, you have an obvious pathophysiology. A blocked blood vessel in the heart due to atherosclerosis leads to chest pain; heart muscle dies; and the patient develops certain symptoms and signs such as chest pain, and shortness of breath. If the patient has pneumonia, the pathophysiology is also clear: an infectious agent has invaded the lung tissue, causing inflammation of the lung and the patient's symptoms.

But what if a patient with chest pain and shortness of breath, doesn't have a heart attack or pneumonia? In this more difficult case, what is the pathophysiology? Is there some rarer infectious or immunologic process that has led to what you see? First, in this type of case, you have to decide if the target of the illness is the heart or the lung. If it's the heart, is the condition due to involvement of the blood vessels of the heart or the heart tissue directly? Is it a viral infection of the heart muscle or a non-infectious inflammation due to immunologic disease of the blood vessels to the heart?

Similarly, if the primary organ affected is the lung, and it's not an obvious pneumonia, I would ask if the cause is vascular, like a pulmonary embolus (blood clot) or an aneurysm (abnormal blood vessels), or a problem with the lung tissue itself ? Again, is it infectious or immunologic? Is it a blood disease in which there is invasion of the lung and/or its blood vessels by leukemia or lymphoma?

In difficult cases, are there any new telltale physical findings that I haven't looked for carefully enough? For example, lymph glands in strange places, like the elbow region, or bleeding (petechiae) in the fingernails, that may be telltale clues to specific unusual conditions. Do my available laboratory tests provide new clues? What additional tests can I do now to arrive at a proper diagnosis? Must I biopsy something? You must now search your mental computer's list of possible causes of the patient's illness again and either rule them in for your patient or rule them out. That is the process of "differential diagnosis."

A patient with nausea, vomiting and abdominal pain will usually undergo an upper GI series of x-rays and an endoscopy, a visual inspection of the stomach and duodenal area, to rule out an ulcer. But if there is no ulcer or other disease seen with these tests, then other laboratory tests will be necessary to rule out rarer metabolic, inherited or infectious causes of the patient's symptoms. The pain, nausea and vomiting may be coming from stimulation of the patient's nerve centers controlling these symptoms. The patient with nausea, vomiting and abdominal pain can also theoretically have Addison's disease, adrenal insufficiency, the disease John F. Kennedy suffered with undiagnosed for many years. Or acute intermittent porphyria, a rare inherited disease with which these symptoms are associated. A simple urinary porphyrin test can establish the diagnosis, and there are drug and dietary treatments for the disease. On the other hand, the patient with the same symptoms may have an adrenal tumor, a pheochromocytoma, and, again, certain special blood tests can establish this diagnosis and lead to successful treatment. We have to be thorough enough and compulsive enough to diagnose these rare causes of common symptoms, especially when these diagnoses can lead to effective treatment.

If tests on the patient with nausea and vomiting reveal that he or she is bleeding from the gastrointestinal tract, we must quickly find out exactly where in the GI tract the bleeding is occurring. Endoscopy of the upper and lower GI tract usually provides the location and cause of the bleeding. Is there an ulcer, a tumor, or deranged blood vessels? If all are negative, then perhaps the bleeding is due to a blood disorder that is causing defective blood clotting, and that is the pathophysiology of the blood loss. Appropriate tests can make that diagnosis, if the clinician thinks of it.

Physicians must always be sure that the routine tests were properly done. For example, in a patient with obvious upper gastrointestinal bleeding, was the endoscopy properly done? Was it indeed truly negative for an ulcer, the most common cause. I remember a ward patient of mine who we thought for sure was bleeding from a stomach ulcer, but who had three negative endoscopies by a GI fellow and attending at the time. The ulcer was finally found at a fourth endoscopy by a competent GI attending after I convinced him personally to do it again. We just couldn't believe the negative results. The lesson here is that if you as the physician believe in a specific diagnosis, you may have to work extra hard to get your subspecialist colleagues to confirm or rule out the diagnosis with certainty.

It is critically important to rule out certain serious and treatable illnesses in every case. After complete evaluation of any patient, you may be left without a specific diagnosis, but the very least we must do as physicians is to rule out serious treatable illness. For example, if a patient has chest pain, we must rule out a heart attack or bacterial pneumonia; and if there is GI bleeding, we must rule out an ulcer or tumor. At the same time, we are constantly searching for alternative diagnoses, if these relatively common and serious conditions do not explain the patient's symptoms and signs and the symptoms and signs do not spontaneously subside.

Sometimes, even the best of us will be fooled by following the most logical path to a diagnosis, and neglect to rule out all of the obvious alternatives. I still remember one case from my days as an intern at Boston City Hospital in which I was terribly mistaken in my judgment.

A man with documented liver disease, cirrhosis, came in with increasing jaundice and evidence of an acute infection. We thought his symptoms were typical for advanced active liver disease due to alcohol, alcoholic cirrhosis. All of his laboratory tests were consistent with that diagnosis, but he did not respond well to antibiotics and supportive care. His jaundice continued to worsen and he finally died.

At autopsy, in addition to alcoholic cirrhosis, he was found to have gallstones (that were not visible by x-ray) and a ruptured gall bladder that we had not diagnosed or thought about seriously. The diagnosis and prompt treatment of the gall bladder disease could have saved this patient's life, at least for a while longer. We should have done tests to rule out the presence of treatable gall bladder disease even though we had an explanation for his symptoms and signs in his liver abnormalities.

Much more recently, a friend of mine became ill with right upper quadrant pain. He had known gall bladder disease and had been asymptomatic for several years. With a recent episode of right-sided abdominal pain typical of gall bladder disease, it was decided that he should finally have gall bladder surgery. At surgery, a relatively rare malignant tumor of the gall bladder was found in addition to his gallstones. He died of the spread of the tumor during the next year despite extensive radiotherapy and chemotherapy. Who knows whether he would have been cured or his life prolonged if he had had his gall bladder surgery earlier and the smaller tumor removed then, if his doctors or I, his friend, had pushed for him to do so?

The main goals in the care of any patient are to establish a diagnosis, and to begin appropriate treatment once the diagnosis is established or after appropriate tests have been done. You don't necessarily need a firm diagnosis to institute emergency treatment but you should have one before definitive treatment. In a patient bleeding from GI disease, we can give blood transfusions without a diagnosis being established if the bleeding is severe enough and there are symptoms from it. Similarly, as mentioned earlier, if someone has a fever and evidence of infection, you want to take samples of blood and fluids — sputum if there's lung disease, or urine if there's evidence for kidney or bladder disease — before instituting antibiotic therapy. You can always change the antibiotic, if the cultures show that you have chosen the wrong one for the particular pathogen.

The Ward Service team, including house officers and attendings like me at Columbia-Presbyterian, took care of patients on the general medical wards, and were particularly secure in taking care of difficult or complicated cases. We knew that if we were unsure of the diagnosis and treatment of particular cases, we had the strong back-up of subspecialists who were more knowledgeable than we were about the particular case at hand and who were immediately available to us.

In addition, medical subspecialists were often consulted even when we, the ward team, had made the diagnosis and instituted treatment. This was to verify that we, the ward team, had instituted the proper treatment plan; to share information and exposure to specific cases with the subspecialists; and to determine who would follow specific patients once they left the hospital. We, the ward team, were, after all, a teaching service. However, we didn't want to waste other people's time with excessive consults, so we picked our occasions for consultation carefully.

During the early days of my career, there were relatively rudimentary special areas in hospitals for either emergency or subspecialty care. Later on, and today, there are highly sophisticated units specializing in intensive care; cardiac intensive care units; cancer wards; special areas for seriously ill patients with infectious communicable diseases; and large Emergency Departments. Extremely ill patients are much more likely to be admitted to these special units today. As a result of these changes, today's Ward Service is more likely to contain patients with diagnostic problems and less likely to house severely ill patients. The exposure of house staff to the whole array of sick patients today will depend on rotations through the special units. This is in contrast to my earlier days on the medical wards at the Boston City Hospital and Presbyterian Hospital when, at any minute of the day, I might be confronted with primary responsibility for a very sick patient needing urgent or very specialized care.

CHAPTER NINE

Columbia-Presbyterian Medicine

In my life in medicine, I have not experienced the intensely demanding life of a private practitioner continually taking care of private patients. I have practiced medicine in a different way, as an academic physician, without the stresses and pressures of today's, or even yesterday's, practicing physicians. I have a relatively short emotional fuse, and given the complexities and abusive machinations of the insurance industry over the years, I may not have responded well. The constant pressures of the private practice of patient care at its best might well be more than I could have handled full-time for any sustained period of my life. I certainly would have been hard pressed to handle the pressures of internists in private practice today.

On the other hand, although I have primarily been involved in medical research in my career, for over 40 years, I have never stopped teaching and seeing patients in teaching and care settings in the hospital, and helping people with their medical problems in and out of the hospital. More specifically, I have been an internist, hematologist and teacher at Columbia-Presbyterian Medical Center (CPMC), now, New York-Presbyterian Hospital. I cared for patients at CPMC as part of my responsibilities as a faculty member in the Department of Medicine starting in 1964 and continuing until my retirement in 2005. I moved up the academic ladder to become a full Professor of Medicine in 1978, and I was Director of the Division of Hematology from 1980 to 2005. I estimate that I spent close to 20% of my professional time in the practice of medicine taking care of patients.

I have always thought of myself as a good doctor because I have always believed I was offering the best medical advice and care available to my patients. Whenever I have seen patients, even casually, my only concern has been for them. I always left my ego outside the room. I think my patients have always trusted me and believed that my sole focus was on them. I have also always recognized when I needed the help of other physicians to take care of specific problems of my patients that I could not handle myself, and, as a result, my patients had confidence that I would do so when the need arose.

Whenever I worked with other physicians, I always felt it was important for me to express my opinions fully, especially if I disagreed with their medical care, but I never tried to change the attitudes of doctors I worked with in any formal way. Actually, I think that most doctors are pretty set in their ways of interacting with patients by their personalities and experiences early in their careers, and that these attitudes are difficult to change. With physicians in training, I tried to teach my ways of interacting with patients by example; I was always aware that it was by example that I had learned about the doctor-patient relationship during my medical training at the Boston City Hospital as well as from people I was exposed to at Columbia-Presbyterian, like Dr. Leifer, really extraordinarily understanding and caring physicians all. I tried to communicate my own personal approach to patient care mainly at the bedside of patients, and primarily to house officers.

I learned a lot about doctor-patient relationships when I was a patient. I saw the doctors' attitudes that I liked and didn't like first hand. Calmness, gentleness, directness as well as expertise in doctors were the main positive ingredients. I think that the Golden Rule is most instructive: To treat patients the way you would want to be treated as a patient yourself.

Throughout my career, I was always a Columbia-Presbyterian employee, and, as it happens, I don't remember ever submitting a bill for my private consultation services to any patient directly. I engaged in five types of medical activities as a physician: (1) caring for patients hospitalized on the wards of Presbyterian Hospital (ward rounds); (2) caring for patients in general medical clinic (out-patient medical clinic); (3) caring for patients hospitalized with hematology or oncology problems as in-patients (hematology-oncology rounds); (4) caring for patients in the out-patient hematology clinic (out-patient hematology clinic); and (5) consulting on patients in hematology conferences at Columbia-Presbyterian while head of the Division of Hematology.

In all of these roles, I was a teacher of medical students, house staff and other physicians, as well as a caregiver to patients.

Ward Rounds

My most intensive experiences in medicine occured while making rounds on the general medical wards at CPMC, which I did from 1965 to 2000. Every year, I spent one month on the medical wards of Presbyterian Hospital. For six or seven days a week I was overseeing the care of general medical patients with severe illnesses in all fields of internal medicine. These patients had no private physician, only house officers (house staff), interns and residents (now called PG1 or PG-2, etc.). I was their senior physician and felt responsible for their care.

These rounds involved seeing these sick hospitalized patients in a "teaching setting" with house staff and medical students, and occasionally other visitors. I, the "ward attending" was, however, not only a teacher, but also one of the two senior physicians, responsible for the care of patients on a particular medical ward. Of course, the house staff wrote the orders, monitored the patients from minute to minute, and were their more immediate physicians. But I felt as personally responsible for the care of every patient I saw on the medical wards as I would have if they were private patients of mine.

Every new patient that had been admitted the day and night before was presented in great detail by a house officer the next day. We usually met for two hours from ten to noon in an alcove or meeting room of some type on the medical floor on which we were making rounds. Before 1984, in the old Presbyterian Hospital building near Broadway and 168th Street; after that, in the newer Milstein Pavilion on Fort Washington Avenue.

There was no course given to me in or after medical school on how to make ward rounds. I had learned how to do so through internalizing examples from my own experiences as a house officer at the Boston City Hospital on the Harvard II and IV Medical Service in the early '60s. I continued to learn how to make rounds when I came to PH from people like Ed Leifer. Most patients I saw on the PH wards were admitted to the hospital after having been seen in the emergency room by other physicians. These were patients who were deemed to be too sick or too difficult to diagnose and treat as outpatients. Thus, only seriously ill patients or those with diagnostic problems were admitted to the wards.

On ward rounds at PH, there were usually two to four house officers as well as two to four medical students, the "medical team." The cases were formally presented by a house officer or medical student, in a room that we could commandeer, or in an alcove or veranda if we could not find a room, and the diagnostic possibilities and treatment up to that point were reviewed. Each new case discussion usually took 20 to 30 minutes.

On rounds, I tried to create an atmosphere in which everyone — students, interns, residents, and co-attendings — felt free to express their thoughts about the patient and the case. While the presentations were fairly formal, I always hoped the overall atmosphere was informal and relaxed. No one was pressured. Anyone could ask a question at any time although we had to try to keep the rounds moving. After the formal presentation of the case was over, and before we discussed the patient's further diagnostic workup and treatment more fully, the whole team (students, house staff, and co-attendings) went to meet and examine the patient.

I preferred not to have the formal presentation of the patient's history, physical findings, lab results, and medical evaluation take place at the patient's bedside, as some other physicians did. I always thought that approach was too invasive of the patient's privacy. The team was a large group of people, largely unknown to the patient. I felt it often either embarrassed or frightened the patient to see us all marching in together.

I thought that the presentation of the case was an academic and teaching exercise as well as one of clinical care, and that the discussion of the case was done more completely and critically away from the patient. Presenting the case at the patient's bedside would make me feel constrained in my questioning of the students and house staff. I had no problem critiquing the care of the patient with the team away from the bedside, but I felt constricted about doing so at the patient's bedside because it could embarrass the student or house officer, and that was certainly not something I wanted the patient to see.

We routinely had two co-attendings, one academic like me, and the other more clinical, a practitioner. At the bedside, my co-attending and I were introduced to the patient by the house officer who admitted the patient. We were called "attendings" or "senior doctors." If it was my case,

I usually then introduced myself to the patient as Doctor Bank, shook hands and said hello. I always wore a button-down shirt and tie under my white coat when I saw patients. It was my sign of respect. I also always called the patient "Mr" or "Mrs" or "Ms," using their last name unless they were really old acquaintances. I then asked the patient questions in my own words that I thought were critical to the immediate present illness in order to confirm independently what I had been told.

I confirmed the patient's history by asking the patient questions like "What brought you to the hospital?" "How long have you had that?" "How do you feel now?" If I got answers that didn't jibe with what I had heard presented or that suggested new avenues of diagnosis to pursue, I would expand my questioning then and there. In this visit, I acted as if I, and the team, had all the time in the world to be with the patient. I tried to project the image to patients that I was interested in nothing else in the world at that time but them, no matter how short or long a time I spent at the bedside. They, the patients, were the reason for my being there.

I then usually did a physical exam to confirm the staff's major positive findings, if any. In addition, I would almost always feel the patients' pulse; look at their skin and eyes; listen to their lungs and heart; feel the abdomen for masses or enlarged organs; look at their legs for edema. I would point out any new physical findings I discovered to the students and house staff at the bedside, if I found significant ones; I would not further question the students or house staff or discuss the patient at the bedside.

There were usually two to four new cases each day, and other sick patients who needed our follow-up every day. If there were too many new patients to be seen on rounds on any given day, I would abbreviate the bedside visit with a hello and very quick appraisal, and tell the patient that I would be back later to talk to them and to examine them more fully, which I did.

After seeing and examining a new patient, the entire medical team including the other attending and myself would retreat to our room or our corner of the hall to review the major points of the cases briefly, and then discuss appropriate further tests and treatment, adding to our thinking what we had learned at the bedside. Again, away from the patient.

The intern was the doctor in charge on an ongoing basis of every case at PH, and we always let the intern on his or her own transmit our advice to the patient. When I was the attending, this was again done out of the sight of the team. On rare occasions, when indicated, I would discuss the case alone with the patient, at the bedside, or with the intern present, especially if the patient or the intern requested it. I felt my main job was to be a consultant to the house staff and insure the best care of the patient. I wrote an "Attending Note" in the official hospital chart on every patient admitted to my care, and follow-up notes during the patient's hospitalization.

Other attendings at PH would do more teaching at the bedside but I always thought that my way was best. Over time, I think the house staff at PH came to know my style. I know that other physicians liked to have more discussion and do more teaching at the bedside, but I do not know to this day why they would want to do so since I think it does not serve the best interests of either the patients or the house staff as individuals to do so. I thought that these discussions, if they were frank and as constructively critical as I always wanted them to be, would, at least on some occasions, negatively affect the relationships that house officers had established with patients, as well as possibly distort the patient's view of what we were thinking. I know that when I was a patient, I would not have appreciated a medical team discussing my case at my bedside. In over 30 years of ward rounds, I never had a co-attending dispute how much (or little) teaching we did at the patient's bedside. I don't know whether this was because they conformed out of respect for me or because they all in fact agreed with me.

I was all business on ward rounds when the medical team was outside of earshot of the patients. I asked tough questions and did not hesitate to indicate to house staff or medical students when I thought they should have done more or different things in their work-up of patients: in taking the history; in doing the physical; in ordering emergency lab tests; in scheduling tests to confirm their diagnostic suspicions; in instituting emergency therapy; in devising a short-term and a long-term plan.

I was not a touchy-feely attending. I was there to teach the students and house staff the right way to do medicine. In my world, there was always a right way to do medicine, and I wanted them to be exposed to it.

With a young, relatively inexperienced ward team, there were, of course, doctor-patient interactions that had to be monitored and edited whenever necessary. The PH house staff was generally quite sensitive to patients' feelings. There were only a few egregious things that I remember seeing on my watch at the bedside. Once, relatively early on in my career, our ward team was at the bedside of a patient, and one of the residents suddenly began to explain the patient's illness to the patient in front of all of us. He said: "Your heart is very flabby. It's like a big bag filled with fluid that isn't pumping well. Your lungs are filling up with fluid and we're giving you medicine to help you. You're very sick."

I didn't appreciate this resident's outburst at all and told him so, but not at the bedside, only when we were back in our meeting place afterwards discussing the case. I told him about his lack of sensitivity and poor judgment. I made sure the house officer in this particular situation knew that he had done his talking to the patient at the wrong time, and in the wrong way. He should not have done it while others, all of us, the team, were there at the bedside. And in private, or in the presence of one or two of us, when he was talking with the patient, he should have used a more empathetic explanation, something like: "We've found that you're heart isn't working properly (or as strong as it should be). It's enlarged. And we're giving you medicines to make it better."

I confronted and, if necessary, admonished students and house officers if I thought their reasoning was defective or their attitude toward patients was inappropriate, although it was sometimes painful for them. I was somewhat gentler with students than with house staff. And I really didn't care what they thought about me personally for doing so. I don't think I received very high marks as a house staff or student favorite. I was never trying to become one. I think it is absolutely critical in medical education that house officers and students be aware of when they are wrong in their care of medical patients or in their decorum in medical situations.

I am very proud of the care given to patients at Presbyterian Hospital during my tenure there. I thought the Columbia-Presbyterian ward medical care system was optimal for patient care. There was a two attending system, usually combining a private practitioner like Ed Leifer and a full-time Columbia faculty member, an MD doing research in a medical subspecialty, like me; this system gave the attendings, the supervising team, different views from different physicians. For me, it was a marvelously successful system in which to practice medicine, take care of patients, teach house staff, and learn from others. The house staff and attendings shared responsibility for patient care. I thought the two attendings learned from each other, at least I always did.

The hospital was reimbursed by government for house staff salaries and benefits. During this time, there was also enough money being made by the private physicians in their practices so that they could give a significant amount of time to teaching on the wards without charge. Also, most of the medical staff, all with appointments at Columbia University as well as Presbyterian Hospital, wanted to teach and learn, and the ward experience provided that opportunity.

There was also enough money to support us full-time faculty members without additional remuneration from the hospital or University for our ward duties. And the hospitals were making money through their tertiary care services. So everyone was happy.

For the most part, everyone who walked through the doors of the hospital or into its emergency room was taken care of promptly and well. Very few patients were turned away. There were stories when I arrived at PH in 1964 of patients who, after being seen in the ER, were put in taxis and were sent to other hospitals as undesirable or non-paying patients, but I never saw any of that activity. Medicare came into existence in 1965 and with more Federal reimbursement, rules for care in hospitals receiving Federal support became more stringent.

Presbyterian Hospital was making money in the '60s through the '80s largely as a tertiary care center and there was no pressure to turn anyone away, whether the person could afford care or not. In addition, physician services to the poor and others without private insurance were given on the hospital wards largely pro bono by the private physicians at Presbyterian Hospital and by people like me who were full-time Columbia faculty; it was part of our jobs as full-time faculty at Columbia University.

General Medical Clinic

I also attended general medical clinic at Columbia-Presbyterian for many years, essentially volunteering to do this service with no remuneration, just because I liked it and wanted to continue to see general medical cases, although I was also by then fully ensconced in hematology and oncology. The patients I saw in general medical clinic were mostly those seen in general medical practice, with common medical diseases such as diabetes, hypertension, arteriosclerotic heart disease and congestive failure.

There were also some diagnostic workups to be done on new patients. I enjoyed that activity as well. For example, I always did testing of new patients with hypertension for the possibility that they had rare causes of their hypertension, such as pheochromocytomas (adrenal tumors); kidney disease; or other endocrine causes. I called it "going once around the block" in my work-up of any new patient.

It has been a long time since I have kept up with all of the advances in diagnosis and treatment that one must be aware of if one is to be an effective general practitioner or general internist today. There are new diagnostic tests; new antibiotics; new anti-hypertensive medications; and many other new treatments for many diseases. These advances constitute today's bread and butter knowledge that general practitioners and internists must continue to acquire to provide up to date care to patients.

I do think, however, that my training and long active medical experience have allowed me to continue to be a fairly competent diagnostician over these many years, even outside my subspecialty. Diagnostic criteria have not changed much over the past fifty years. My continued interest in patient care and my general medical knowledge and (I think) good medical judgment are qualities that have endured, despite the passing of time. Now that I'm retired, I still feel confident in assessing medical problems brought to my attention, and referring patients to appropriate internists and specialists I know and trust.

CHAPTER TEN

Becoming a Hematologist

My subspecialty

In addition to being trained in general internal medicine, I am also trained as a hematologist, and have practiced this subspecialty for over 40 years. After medical school and house staff training and two years of research at the National Institutes of Health (NIH), I became a hematology fellow at Columbia-Presbyterian in 1964. After my fellowship training, I became a full-time faculty member at Columbia University and became Board certified in hematology. I was a hematology consult and made rounds on patients with hematological diseases on the wards of Presbyterian Hospital one or two months a year. These were sub-specialty rounds, separate from my general ward rounding responsibilities. I consulted on patients with all kinds of hematological problems hospitalized on the general medical wards and on the more specialized cancer wards when they were established later on.

As part of my clinical responsibilities, I also attended a hematology out-patient clinic one afternoon a week from 1964 to 2000, seeing several patients a day. I was director of the Division of Hematology in the Department of Medicine at Columbia-Presbyterian from 1980 to 2005. During that time, I also led a weekly Thursday morning two-hour hematology conference, attended by both full-time faculty in hematology and private practitioners, in which both private and ward cases were reviewed. Although the conference was mainly focused on teaching, it was quite relevant to patient care as well. As head of hematology I felt it was my responsibility to chair the conference. I also hosted guest lecturers who spoke about research or clinical topics in hematology at weekly conferences Thursday afternoons.

A new life

I arrived at my decision to become a hematologist while completing my military service requirement as a research associate in the United States Public Health Service (USPHS) at the NIH between 1962 and 1964. During this time, and surprisingly to me, I fell in love with laboratory research. Until then, I thought my future would be solely in the private practice of internal medicine. I had just completed two years of internship and residency in internal medicine at the Boston City Hospital and was prepared for and excited about a career as a practitioner of internal medicine. But going to the NIH was also an opportunity for me to try to do basic laboratory research in-depth, something I had not done before.

I was fortunate to find a research opportunity at the NIH in 1962. The NIH is the jewel in the crown of American medical research. It is a shining example of the ability of government in the United States to create programs of excellence in areas critical to the public interest, in this case, science and medicine, when it is committed to do so. The United States has the best and most productive scientific community in the world because of our government's funding through the NIH of basic and clinical research at universities throughout the country, as well as at the NIH campus in Bethesda, Maryland. The US Congress should be extolled for its creation and continued support of the NIH.

The process of devising experiments and physically performing them to ask and answer basic scientific questions was new to me when I arrived at the NIH. But while I was there, it became rapidly clear to me that this activity in basic research was going to continue for me and was going to be a major part of my professional life. At the NIH, I worked on the role of a specialized RNA, soluble or transfer RNA, one of the many molecules involved in synthesizing proteins. The project and experiments I did at this time had no clear relevance to human biology or medicine, but they provided me with an in-depth experience of what true basic laboratory research was and how it was done.

I was fortunate to have three PhD mentors at the NIH who were all excellent scientists: Drs. Alan Peterkofsky, Alan Mehler and Fred Bergmann. I learned from all of them. They taught me how to think about an experiment; then devise it; then carry it out and interpret the results. My experience at the NIH changed the course of my professional life.

As it turned out, I discovered that I was a good scientist. I had always been curious about the details of new things I had learned in school and in medicine. I had an open mind. I thought logically. I was imaginative. In fact, during the ensuing 40-plus years in research I never had a moment when I felt I didn't know the next logical experiment to do on any given research project. I was patient and seldom confounded by the twists and turns of scientific discovery. I succeeded in research with confidence until I retired.

Science captivated me. I loved everything about the process of investigating a problem on my own: obsessing about how to solve a problem, and devising and carrying out experiments to do so, even if a medically meaningful positive result was years away.

I have written a book, *Turning Blood Red: The Fight for Life in Cooley's Anemia*, (World Scientific Publications, 2009) which discusses the research that I did in over 40 years at Columbia on the molecular biology of hemoglobin, and its role in a human genetic blood disease, beta thalassemia. As detailed in the book, I worked primarily on understanding what caused beta thalassemia at the molecular level, and on trying to find unique approaches, such as gene therapy, to treating the disease. About 80% of my time was devoted to research, and the rest was as a clinician doing medicine and engaged in the specialty of hematology.

It was a particular honor and privilege for me to be an independently funded American scientist for five decades. I answered to no one as long as I succeeded in obtaining NIH funding from research grants, which I did continuously from 1964 to 2009. I had freedom in the lab: I could do the experiments I wanted to do; hire the people I wanted to work with; and pursue my research life with no one telling me what I had to do. I could be thinking or doing science 24/7 or not; it was my choice. I could be as selfish as I wanted with my thoughts, and as self-centered as I wanted with my actions, my time, my research money, as long as they were in the service of my scientific goals. There are few other careers like it.

It is, however, a scary experience to depend on successfully competing for research grants every three to five years in order to continue to be a self-sustaining academic physician-scientist. Success or failure is completely based on the recommendation of a peer review grant committee evaluating your research and deciding whether you are worthy of continuing support.

I, like most researchers, had no back-up sources of research funding if all of my NIH research applications were unfunded. Therefore, I always had two or three research projects in progress so that I could withstand the fiscal consequences if one application on a given project was rejected. Being judged on every new or renewal grant application was always a traumatic experience, although success made the process worthwhile. Many scientists fall by the wayside over time in this competitive process and then go on to do other things. When they do, PhDs most often go to work for drug companies or teach, and MDs either go into private practice or teach or go to work for drug companies or HMOs. Much of my Columbia University salary was paid for by my research grants so I was not particularly beholden to income from my clinical activities to support myself.

Making another decision

While at the NIH, I decided that laboratory research would be a large part of my future career. I also decided I wanted to be a clinical hematologist, a blood specialist, as well as an internist. Hematology is the subspecialty of medicine that deals with the blood system. Blood cells are made in the bone marrow, spaces within our bones, filled with cells and fat. The blood cells produced in the bone marrow spaces include red blood cells; white blood cells, lymphocytes and granulocytes; and platelets. Red blood cells contain hemoglobin, a protein that carries oxygen to our tissues; white blood cells combat infectious agents; and platelets help our blood to clot. All of the cells of the blood (or hematopoietic) system originate from a small number of extra-special cells called blood stem cells in the bone marrow.

The field of hematology encompasses the normal and abnormal development of all blood cells. The major hematologic diseases are: (1) the anemias, due to abnormal or decreased red blood cells; (2) leukemias, lymphomas and multiple myeloma, due to problems with white blood cells; and (3) the thrombocytopenias or platelet problems, and other bleeding defects like hemophilia. Blood banking, stem cell biology and bone marrow transplantation are also in the purview of hematology.

The field of hematology has grown and expanded enormously during the past half-century. Our understanding of diseases of the blood today, of their diagnosis and treatment, in no way resembles what we knew or had available to us when I entered the field in the 1960s. Every aspect of the biology and pathology of blood and bone marrow function and dysfunction has been studied intensively since then, and the cellular and molecular events occurring normally and in diseases have been clarified. We now know the causes and pathophysiology of most anemias, both inherited and acquired. Abnormal genetic events of many kinds have been found to cause anemias, leukemias and lymphomas, and platelet diseases as well. The biology of proteins, such as erythropoietin, granulocyte-stimulating factors, thrombopoietin and other growth factors, necessary for blood stem cells to evolve into all of our blood cell elements has been elucidated.

Life at the NIH

I wanted to continue to see patients as part of my career even though I was increasingly becoming interested in research. While at the NIH, I became intrigued with hematology as a potential medical subspecialty. There were many reasons for choosing hematology although even today I don't clearly have them in order of their importance to me. One reason was certainly the emergence of exciting new technologies that I learned to use in my laboratory work at the NIH in the early 1960s; I could see these advances in molecular biology being applied to the study of blood and human disease. I could also see that being a hematologist could allow me to combine a career in clinical medicine with laboratory research. I began to think about studying human hemoglobin, the major protein in red blood cells that carries oxygen around the body, as a potential major focus of my future research.

I also learned a lot about the nuts and bolts of a career in clinical hematology at the NIH. Dr. George Brecher, chief of the hematology section of the Department of Clinical Pathology at NIH at the time, assisted me greatly in thinking about a career in clinical hematology and, more importantly, exposing me to, and teaching me about, blood and bone marrow morphology. I spent hours in my spare time looking through the microscope at blood and bone marrow specimens with Dr. Brecher as he was reviewing material from patients, mainly children with acute leukemia, who were being treated on the clinical wards at the NIH. He showed me how to systematically examine the blood and marrow for different cell types of normal blood cells; to identify their characteristics; and to ascertain their specific abnormal diagnostic features in disease. These were lessons I would never forget.

Hematology also appealed to me since it was one of the few medical specialties that, even in the 1960s, offered the availability of effective therapies for many of its diseases. Even in those early days, safe blood transfusions were available that could benefit, if not cure, many anemias. Also many new chemotherapeutic agents were just being developed to treat patients with leukemias and lymphomas.

Several of my colleagues at the NIH were Clinical Associates in the National Cancer Institute who were involved in clinical trials of drugs in treating children with acute leukemia. Most of these Associates did not go into hematology because of the extreme emotional trauma they experienced treating very sick young children with very toxic experimental drugs that caused severe clinical side effects. Although these treatments cured some of those children, many others succumbed to their disease. I don't know if I would have become a clinical hematologist if I had been similarly engaged in caring for these sick children, even if I believed what turned out to be true: that treatments initiated at the NIH at the time would lead to the discovery of more effective drug regimens for the treatment of children and adults with leukemia.

Returning to Columbia

Having made the choice to specialize in hematology at the NIH, I had to decide where to do a hematology fellowship and continue my clinical and research training. The best acknowledged clinical hematology programs were in Salt Lake City, Utah, Washington University in St. Louis, and the University of Washington in Seattle, but I decided to go back to my hometown, New York City.

I looked at several excellent hematology programs in the city, including Mount Sinai, Albert Einstein, NYU and Columbia-Presbyterian. With my interest in hematology research, I initially favored the Einstein program because of the presence of Dr. Helen Ranney. She was an outstanding clinician and research hematologist, the kind I wanted to be. She worked on the structure and function of human hemoglobin, the protein in which I was most interested. With new emerging technologies, there were many new questions to be addressed in Dr. Ranney's laboratory about hemoglobin's complex role in health and disease. But when I interviewed with her and informed her of my interest in molecular biology, Dr. Ranney urged me to consider Columbia's hematology program where Dr. Paul Marks was working in the area of protein synthesis that I seemed to be focused on pursuing. She knew the program well as she had previously been on the faculty at Columbia.

I stayed in touch with Helen Ranney throughout my career. She was an extraordinary person, clinician and scientist. She later headed west to be the first woman to head a department of medicine in the United States at UCSF and she became a leader in American medicine. We always had a good laugh together, and enjoyed each other's company at national meetings. I remember once, in later years, we shared teaching assignments on the Education Program of the national meeting of the American Society of Hematology. Dr. Ranney was to discuss sickle cell anemia and I thalassemia. After we had given our talks for the first time and were waiting to repeat them to a new audience, she said. "Wanna switch? You talk about sickle; I'll talk about thal," while delighting me with her characteristic cackling laugh. It was hard to refuse her request, but I did so, fearing that I would embarrass myself by my relatively lesser mastery of both content and presentation in talking about sickle cell anemia. Helen was game for anything.

I decided to become a hematology fellow at Columbia in 1964 and never regretted my choice. The reputation of Columbia-Presbyterian as a superb medical training institution also influenced me. I enjoyed returning to New York after an eight-year absence. I had never worked at Presbyterian Hospital (PH), part of Columbia-Presbyterian Medical Center (CPMC), but I had great respect for its clinical and scientific reputation. However, while I was happy to be there, I was not in awe of my new professional home. I had been well-trained at Harvard Medical School, the Boston City Hospital and the NIH and I was confident of my abilities.

The hematology service at Columbia-Presbyterian in 1964 was miniscule; it consisted of a small room on the 8th floor of the College of Physicians and Surgeons (P&S), which doubled as a special clinical hematology lab. The fellows occupied part of the room. Ms. Sylvia Ford, a laboratory technician of long-standing at that time (she later went on to medical school), was the power behind the throne. She was the head of the special hematology laboratory, part of the clinical laboratories of the hospital, and she did all the special tests on patient material like hemoglobin analyses, special blood enzyme tests and other blood analyses. Dr. Marks' research laboratories were in a separate space, on the 12th floor of a connected building, Vanderbilt Clinic.

The primary duty of the clinical fellow as in most clinical hematology programs was to respond to requests for hematology consults from the ward services. I had never worked at a New York hospital before nor had I ever before been involved with consulting on tertiary care patients. The experience was new to me. I hadn't really been exposed to much clinical hematology in my house staff training at the Boston City Hospital. Not that many patients with hematological problems were admitted there. Most of the patients I saw had common medical diseases like pneumonia, alcoholism, heart attacks, bleeding ulcers and the like. Folic acid deficiency associated with alcoholism was the most common hematological disorder I remember seeing at the BCH.

I was most immediately impressed with both the quality of the physicians I met at PH and the medical records of the patients. I was actually enchanted to read the written record of each patient, many of whom had been cared for at the institution for many years. The thoroughness, clarity and availability of the medical records at PH amazed me. It was like reading a non-fiction book in all of its details, and I liked details. It was a far cry from my experience at the BCH where charts were sometimes incomplete and often difficult to find. I was also impressed with the variety of patients seen at PH and their complex problems; diseases like lupus, hemophilia, sickle cell disease, leukemia, lymphoma. Patients with these conditions were much more common at PH than at the BCH.

Don't get me wrong. The two years I spent at the BCH taught me all I really needed to know about how to take care of very sick patients. Nothing that I encountered in medicine after my internship and year of residency there could overwhelm me. It was just that at BCH as a house officer, I was so busy taking care of my own very sick patients that I had little time to think in depth about most complex medical problems, if and when I did get to see them. Doing hematology at Presbyterian Hospital was more like working as a private physician in a prestigious academic medical center (which PH was and is) with more time to spend seeing patients with complicated illnesses and thinking about their problems.

As I began seeing patients as a clinical hematology fellow at PH, I had much to learn. I had just returned from my two years at the NIH doing research there, with extremely little exposure to clinical medicine during that time. In addition, I didn't know or remember much hematology. I needed a lot of help and I received it. I particularly remember Dr. Helen Anderson as one of the best of the clinical hematologists I worked with during my fellowship and in my early years. Drs. Paul Marks and Richard Rifkind, my lab mates, were also excellent clinical hematology mentors. Drs. George Hyman and Robert Kritzler were additional experienced clinical hematologists who also helped me then.

CHAPTER ELEVEN

Hematology and Oncology

Oncology, the medical sub-specialty concerned with the study of cancer, was in its infancy in the '60s. Hematologic malignancies (cancers) were the joint purview of hematology and oncology. Dr. John Ultmann, an oncologist, was the most prominent specialist taking care of patients with hematologic malignancies at Columbia when I arrived. He was the first oncologist I had ever met. He was based at Delafield Hospital, a city hospital, bordered by Haven Avenue, 165th Street, Riverside Drive and 163rd Street. The hospital has since been demolished and replaced by a parking lot.

Dr. Ultmann, his name appropriate to his demeanor, was an intense, demanding man, and an excellent clinician. He had a clinic population full of patients with lymphomas (cancers of the lymphatic cells) whom he followed closely. They were mainly patients with Hodgkin's disease, and were the relatively rare long-term survivors of the disease in the '60s. Drug therapy (chemotherapy) with steroids, cyclophosphamide, and nitrogen mustard was the mainstay of lymphoma treatment in the early '60s. While some patients with Hodgkin's disease did well with this limited treatment, and some lived long lives, few were cured. These were the days just before the use of more effective, curative combination chemotherapy for the lymphomas with the addition of newer more active drugs, especially the anthracyclines (Daunomycin and Adriamycin), and the vinca alkaloids (vincristine and vinblastine).

We, the fellows, were the beneficiaries of Dr. Ultmann's clinic and his long experience in the diagnosis and treatment of these patients. Dr. Ultmann was an excellent teacher in the European tradition of asking questions and rapidly supplying answers, with little actual dialogue. I never minded the style. I would learn what I needed to learn in any way that was available to me: through monologues from teachers like John Ultmann or dialogues with them. Dr. Ultmann later left Columbia and went on to become head of oncology at the University of Chicago and a prominent national leader in the field.

There were relatively few hematology or oncology fellows in the program at Columbia in the mid '60s. I remember Drs. John Glick and Peter Cassileth who later had successful careers in hematology/oncology at the University of Pennsylvania. Drs. Lionel Grossbard and Bob DeBellis who were fellows with me, stayed on at Columbia.

I was a hematology fellow when the vinca alkaloids were first used at PH. I still remember treating a young man who had Hodgkin's disease involving his bones with vincristine, a newly available drug back then. He was in a single room in the dark wards of the old Presbyterian Hospital, and I gave him his vincristine by vein, the only acceptable route of administration for the drug. He had been unresponsive to the other chemotherapeutic drugs we had tried and I was optimistic that he might respond to the new medicine. What I remember most vividly to this day was how very sad and disappointed I was when the vincristine didn't help and the patient died soon afterwards. He was one of the first young adults I had treated for cancer, and I was especially emotionally affected by his demise. I was frustrated and upset that my treatment had failed. But I told myself then and subsequently that no one else could have done more for him. If I thought someone else or someplace else could have done more, I would have sent my patient to that other physician or facility for care. That's the way I felt back then, and that's the way I felt throughout my career.

Divisions

In the 1960s, there were conflicts between the divisions of hematology and oncology at many hospitals with regard to the responsibility for care of patients with hematologic malignancies: leukemias, lymphomas, myeloma. Hematology divisions at that time were well-established. Oncology divisions were more ill-defined at many institutions. The Division of Oncology at Columbia-Presbyterian, led by Dr. Alfred Gellhorn, was small, even though 25% to 35% of patients admitted to the hospital had a diagnosis of cancer, usually lung, breast or colon cancer.

At many hospitals, there was (and in some cases, still is) a competition for responsibility for the care and treatment of patients with hematologic malignancies: the "blood cancers." These were so-called "liquid tumors" as opposed to breast, lung, etc. cancers which were labeled "solid tumors." Oncologists, whether trained in hematology or not, usually wanted control of the care of patients with hematologic malignancies since these were the patients whose cancers were most treatable and often curable back then and even today.

The guidelines for who controls the care of any given patient with a specific medical diagnosis have always been murky. Certainly, any doctor can legally care for any patient, including those with a diagnosis of cancer, as inexpert as that care might be. And most medical institutions do not monitor the quality of that care by individual physicians.

Most divisions of medical oncology began as groups of subspecialists interested primarily in the non-surgical treatment of cancer patients. After diagnosing colon cancer, most gastroenterologists didn't really want to care for patients with this condition. If the disease was not cured by the surgeons, they, the gastroenterologists, didn't want (and still don't want) responsibility for delivering chemotherapy or radiotherapy. They aren't trained to do so or to handle the side effects of these treatments. Radiation was given by radiation oncologists, and chemotherapy by medical oncologists. Similarly, most pulmonologists (lung specialists), after making the diagnosis of lung cancer, don't want to treat the disease; it is difficult to treat and is most often fatal. Radiotherapy has been somewhat effective and is again given by radiotherapists. Chemotherapy was largely experimental and usually more toxic than effective and was given by medical oncologists. Even today, lung cancer outcomes with chemotherapy are poor.

Most medical subspecialties have a single organ system focus: the heart in cardiology; the GI tract in gastroenterology; the joints and bones in rheumatology, etc. While hematology has always had a clear focus on the blood and bone marrow, the field of oncology has never had such an organ system focus. It has always been more like the study of a collection of a heterogeneous group of diseases to me: cancers of the lung, colon, breast, prostate, brain, have very little in common with each other; and even less with the blood cancers, and so the role of a general medical oncologist has no specific disease system focus.

I always felt that hematology was a coherent medical subspecialty concerned with diseases affecting the cells of the blood and bone marrow. From my earliest days at Columbia-Presbyterian, the Division of Hematology officially controlled the teaching, diagnosis and care of ward patients with leukemias, lymphomas and myeloma. The care of private patients with hematologic malignancies at PH was in the hands of both hematologists and oncologists, some of the latter not specifically trained in hematology. The same situation exists to some extent today. Even as head of the Division of Hematology, and despite my strong feelings that someone with specific training in hematology should care for patients with hematological malignancies, I never could control or monitor the care of all of these patients at PH, especially of private patients.

Today, there are multidisciplinary approaches to treating specific cancers involving medical oncologists, radiotherapists, and surgeons, especially at large medical centers. Organ-specific cancer divisions have been organized to focus on research and treatment of specific tumors. Certainly this is true at Columbia-Presbyterian and has been for a long time, especially in the treatment of genitourinary cancer, and currently of lung, breast and colon cancer.

As I have said before, oncologists have always been especially interested in treating patients with leukemias, lymphomas, and myelomas because even early on, in the '60s and '70s, there were more effective treatments for these cancers than for most solid tumors. National cooperative study groups composed of both hematologists and oncologists were formed to systematically evaluate different treatment regimens for patients with hematological neoplasms, and our division of hematology at Columbia participated in these trials.

In my opinion, the political infighting between separate divisions of hematology and oncology for the control of the care of these patients such as I experienced at Columbia was never on an even playing field. This is primarily because there are so many more patients with solid tumors who are often sicker, particularly with breast, lung and colon cancer, than those with hematological neoplasms. The financial clout of medical oncologists caring for these patients has always resulted in much greater political power in departments of medicine for divisions of oncology than for divisions of hematology. Therefore, there has always been a great deal more money, from private and federal sources, grants and philanthropy by grateful cancer patients, available to divisions of oncology than to divisions of hematology. Also, the establishment of federally funded Comprehensive Cancer Centers, with millions of dollars in grants available, has always been more focused on research, prevention and treatment of solid tumors than of hematological cancers. There has been such a center at Columbia University for many years.

Increased funding for cancer in general from the Federal government, starting with President Nixon's war on cancer in the '70s and continuing into recent decades, led to the building of cancer-specific wards with special sterile facilities for treating patients with very low white blood counts (as a result of chemotherapy) in need of sterile environments. These funds also provided for nurses specifically trained in caring for cancer patients and have resulted in much better care of cancer patients than I received in 1988. Patients with hematologic neoplasms and bone marrow transplantation patients benefited from these units as well, although the units were administered solely by the Oncology Division, not Hematology, at Columbia. With the recent joining of the two divisions into a single Hematology-Oncology Division in 2005, I have heard from my former colleagues that hematologists finally have a seat at the table in discussing overall oncology activities.

Also involved in these political struggles between hematology and oncology was (and is) the control of research and clinical activities in bone marrow transplantation, a treatment that has grown mightily in usage, and, in some circumstances, has generated significant income in departments of medicine over the past 25 years. The chairman of the Department of Medicine was always the ultimate arbiter of these turf wars at CPMC. In my case, the chairmen always came down on the side of oncology: it was a much bigger enterprise and brought in much more money for the Department than hematology. Suffice it to say that I never felt the hematology division had the resources or power to expand its clinical activities at Columbia-Presbyterian in hematologic neoplasms and bone marrow transplantation, or to do new clinical research studies of blood stem cells.

My feeling has always been that because of their training hematologists are more knowledgeable than oncologists without hematological training in understanding and handling the problems of patients with all cancers, not just hematological malignancies; especially the common hematological complications of chemotherapy and the primarily hematological issues inherent in bone marrow transplantation and stem cell therapy. For these reasons, I have always thought that any hematologist could be a good oncologist, but that oncologists not trained in hematology could not handle these problems as well.

Despite the turf battles I fought to try to expand the division of hematology's role, our training program at Columbia-Presbyterian has always been a joint Hematology-Oncology Training Program. Fellows were trained in both hematology and oncology on my watch with only rare exceptions. As I have said, I believe all oncologists should be trained in hematology, and, in order to make a living, hematologists need to see patients with either general medical problems and/or those with solid tumors.

Many fellows in the joint training program were funded by Hematology Training Grants that I generated from NIH to support fellows at Presbyterian from the 1970s until 2002. Thus, I had a major say about which fellows were supported by these training grants. During the last two decades, the fellow pool for our training program has been excellent although fellows interested primarily in hematology and/or in research have been relatively rare. Most graduates want to go into the private practice of oncology, and have done so.

I also insisted that fellows in the training program have at least one year, but more optimally two years, in laboratory research or translational clinical research during their fellowship. I always thought, based on my own experience, that exposure to research contributes to more creative thinking about clinical problems, by honing and enhancing clinical logic and expertise in diagnosis and treatment. I did not allow funds from the Hematology Training Grant to be used to support fellows for clinical training alone.

CHAPTER TWELVE

Doing Hematology

As indicated earlier, hematology is the discipline of studying diseases of the blood and bone marrow, and includes the care of patients with anemias, platelet and coagulation disorders, and hematological neoplasms. Hematologists have always had to be excellent general internists as well. The practice of hematology requires a generalist's approach to many of its patients. The specialty of hematology is unlike those of cardiology or GI where these specialists care for patients with relatively few specific diseases in most of their practice, like coronary artery disease for cardiologists and peptic ulcer disease for GI specialists. Many hematology patients, on the other hand, have diseases involving multiple systems. Anemias can, of course, be due to simple causes like lack of vitamins or iron, but they are often part of more complicated and sometimes esoteric conditions. The hematologist must be familiar with the broad gamut of diseases that can cause anemia, such as rarities like thrombotic thrombocytopenic purpura, a condition which involves blood vessel pathology and is associated not only with anemia, but also thrombocytopenia, kidney disease, and neurologic involvement. Or subacute bacterial endocarditis, an infectious disease caused by heart valve infection, manifesting in anemia, petechiae (skin bleeding), and fever. Or, more commonly, a variety of different infectious, immunologic or oncologic disorders. Similarly, coagulation and bleeding disorders can be due to a wide variety of medical conditions.

The leukemias, lymphomas and myeloma are the glue that holds the discipline of hematology together, combining several elements of blood and bone marrow pathology and problems with systemic disease as well. Patients with these conditions are often the sickest and most challenging in medicine for hematologists. But most patients seen by hematologists have anemia or coagulation or bleeding problems.

Coagulation

Most hematologists take care of all types of hematology patients including those with hematological malignancies; with anemias; and with problems of coagulation, the clotting of blood, and bleeding. As such, I treated many patients with bleeding and coagulation problems, including the most common problem, thrombocytopenia. Thrombocytopenia means reduced platelets. Platelets, cells produced in the bone marrow and then circulated in our blood stream, plug damaged blood vessels when we bleed. Decreased platelets are caused by either decreased platelet production in the bone marrow, or increased platelet destruction in the circulating blood. The most frequent form of thrombocytopenia, immune thrombocytopenia (ITP) in adults, is an immunologically based disorder due to antibodies that result in destruction of platelets. I never became an expert in every disease of coagulation and bleeding, but I became an expert in the care of these patients. If the platelet count is really low, below 20,000, and the patient is bleeding, immediate treatment is necessary to prevent life-threatening bleeding. Corticosteroids and immune gamma globulin usually control the acute form of the disease. Sometimes removal of the spleen (splenectomy) is eventually necessary to normalize the platelet count; the spleen is the most sensitive organ for recognizing and destroying antibody-coated platelets or red cells.

Platelets are one of the components of the blood required for blood clotting; however, there are many proteins, so-called coagulation factors, necessary for this process. Deficiency of certain coagulation factors, factors VIII and IX, are responsible for hemophilia and bleeding. Although I could manage the care of hemophilia patients as a hematology attending if I had to do so, disorders of coagulation were never my forte and are a subspecialty of their own within the specialty of hematology. I was extremely fortunate in having two world experts in coagulation whom I could rely on to help with the special care of these patients at almost all times during my career at CPMC.

Dr. Hymie Nossel was the first of these. He came to CPMC soon after I became an attending physician there, and was an outstanding member of the Department of Medicine until his premature death in 1983. Dr. Nossel made major research contributions to the basic understanding of the delicate balance between bleeding and clotting, and was one of the first scientists to develop special tests to measure the competing actions of two important molecules in this process, plasmin and thrombin.

For his work in this area, Dr. Nossel was world-renowned as a researcher, but he was also an excellent clinical hematologist. Everyone at the medical center called upon him to evaluate and help solve the problems of their patients with coagulation or bleeding issues. All of us at Columbia learned coagulation from Hymie Nossel. But Hymie was much more than an excellent scientist and clinician to many of us. To me personally, he was a good friend and an exceptionally empathetic colleague as well as one of the few physicians or scientists I knew who enjoyed hearing about the success of others in either their professional or personal lives. He also loved to talk about new ideas and was a critical observer of both his own and others' research. He was also a very good listener. There aren't many professional colleagues I have had with whom I have been as close.

Hymie kept himself in splendid physical shape. He was thin and stayed active physically, mainly by running frequently. At age 47, however, one day after running, he collapsed and died suddenly. His death was a shock to all of his family, colleagues and friends. I was heartbroken for the Nossel family and for myself. I still feel sad thinking of his sudden premature death. My wife and I did what we could to keep in touch with his family, including his three young children, at the time and over the subsequent years.

Because of his devotion to science and learning and my personal admiration for him, we established the Hymie Nossel Lectureship in his honor at CPMC. Over the next two decades, we selected the most prominent people in the coagulation field to give these talks. The night of the lectureship was an annual major social occasion for the Division of Hematology, at least I thought so. All of the hematologists in the division, their spouses, and Hymie's wife and children were invited to join with the invited speaker over dinner, usually at the Terrace Restaurant near the Columbia College campus.

Dr. Nossel's death left a major void in clinical expertise and research in coagulation. I finally filled it with the recruitment of Dr. David Diuguid. It was one of the best appointments I ever made. Dr. Diuguid had trained with Drs. Bruce and Barbara Furie, noted coagulation experts, at Tufts University School of Medicine. As well as being an excellent clinician and teacher, David had done laboratory research on the genetic origins of specific coagulation factor deficiencies at Tufts.

Soon after coming to Columbia, Dr. Diuguid not only took the entire medical center's coagulation and bleeding problems on his broad shoulders, he also took on the responsibility of overseeing the special coagulation laboratory. Eventually, because of the press of his clinical and administrative responsibilities, Dr. Diuguid had to end his basic laboratory research program. He has continued to be the star coagulation expert at CPMC for the past two decades, and is currently head of the hematology section in the joint Hematology-Oncology division.

Anemia: the hematologist's forte

Patients with anemia are the mainstay of the practice of hematology. Anemias are diseases with low red blood cell counts, and are caused by decreased production of red blood cells in the bone marrow, by increased destruction of red blood cells in the circulating blood, or by blood loss. Decreased production of red blood cells can be due to deficiencies in substances necessary for normal red cell functioning, like iron, folic acid or vitamin B12, as well as many other causes.

Iron deficiency anemia is the most common anemia by far. While in some underdeveloped countries iron deficiency anemia can be due to dietary deficiency, in the United States iron deficiency anemia is almost always due to bleeding; iron is lost as blood is lost because hemoglobin, the major protein in blood, contains iron. We don't ingest enough iron in our diets to compensate for the iron we lose with significant bleeding. The diagnosis of iron deficiency anemia is made by typical abnormal findings on the blood smear and by blood tests indicating low iron levels.

But iron deficiency anemia, like all anemias, is not really a diagnosis; it is merely a descriptive term; it does not specify a *cause*. In every case of iron deficiency anemia, we need a cause. With menstruation, the cause of iron deficiency anemia is clear, menstrual blood loss, and the patient can be safely treated with iron pills and sent home and followed up appropriately. However, when iron deficiency anemia is found in males or non-menstruating females, it must be explained and a cause must be found. The patient should never be sent home without a diagnosis. A positive test for blood in the stool will focus the physician on the GI tract as the cause of the bleeding. Sometimes, however, the bleeding can be intermittent and a negative test is obtained. GI bleeding is the most common cause of iron deficiency anemia and is usually due to peptic ulcer disease or gastritis, but it can also be due to cancer. When GI bleeding is present in a male or non-menstruating female with iron deficiency anemia the patient needs radiologic and endoscopic evaluation (insertion of a tube for a look-see) of the upper and lower GI tract, gastroscopy and colonoscopy, to rule out stomach or colon cancer and to see if there is an ulcer or gastritis.

The most common medical disaster involving patients with iron deficiency anemia occurs when the physician sends the patient home on iron pills without establishing a cause for the anemia; the iron pills will treat the anemia but the cause, which may be stomach or colon cancer, will remain undetected and may prove fatal. Detection of these cancers, which often can be cured surgically when detected early enough, will be missed, or delayed. I don't know how many times this type of error occurs in the US each year, but I do know personally of several cases in which the cause of iron deficiency anemia was not pursued or a specific diagnosis was made too late to save patients from eventually fatal stomach or colon cancer. This is medical malpractice and, more importantly, has led to unnecessary deaths of patients.

If GI bleeding is absent in a patient with iron deficiency anemia, then other rarer sites for bleeding must be sought, such as urinary or gynecological sources, or even more rarely the lung or other internal organs. Obviously, if the patient has had recent trauma, then bleeding from such a site should be investigated. I once slipped and fell and bled significantly around my hip joint. I never developed anemia. One of my sons developed low iron levels that were detected on blood tests and worried me for a while until I discovered he had donated blood recently.

It does not require a hematologist to diagnose and treat a patient with iron deficiency anemia. But in this rushed world of medicine, if any general practitioner or internist doesn't know the drill in working up an anemia, the physician is best off referring such a patient routinely to a hematologist. Above all, no physician should treat a patient with iron deficiency anemia with iron pills without finding out the cause of the blood loss!

Other causes of anemia can be diagnosed by appropriate special blood tests. Vitamin B12 and folic acid deficiencies due to a variety of causes can be diagnosed in this way. Aplastic anemia is a term applied to anemias in which the marrow produces no or very few red cells. The cause is often unknown. Sometimes anemia is caused by invasion of the marrow by cancer, lymphoma or leukemia. Anemia is also commonly associated with chronic kidney (renal) disease; this anemia is partially due to deficiency of the red cell stimulating hormone, erythropoietin. The availability of the genetically engineered hormone has led to a specific cure.

Often, bone marrow examination is required to arrive at a specific cause for anemia. This requires putting a needle into the bone marrow cavity, usually in the hip area, and withdrawing marrow. Aspiration (pulling out marrow) and biopsy (sampling a piece of the marrow) are not totally innocuous procedures, but in my experience, both should be relatively painless. Using local anesthesia, they are comparable to having a tooth pulled, in my opinion. They shouldn't be more painful than that when done by a competent hematologist.

Anemias can also be due to increased destruction of red blood cells (hemolysis); hemolytic anemias are usually caused by antibodies in the blood that bind to the red blood cells resulting in their premature destruction. Sickle cell disease is another type of hemolytic anemia due to the presence of an abnormal hemoglobin, sickle hemoglobin, that causes the red blood cells to assume an abnormal sickle shape and to be destroyed prematurely. It was the blood disease I treated most often as a hematologist at CPMC, and is the focus of the next chapter.

Determining the underlying cause of the anemia leads to appropriate specific treatment in most cases. Replacement of vitamin B12 or folic acid is the treatment for deficiencies of these vitamins, following a search for specific causes of these deficiencies, usually GI or dietary. Blood transfusions can be used for aplastic anemias and thalassemia; and erythropoietin for the anemia of chronic renal disease. Corticosteroids are used to reduce antibody-mediated destruction of red cells; and splenectomy is used to eliminate the organ most responsible for the premature destruction of antibody-coated red blood cells in certain hemolytic anemias.

Mysteries

While the cause of most anemias becomes clear with a proper evaluation of the patient, there are always a few mysterious unsolved cases. In these cases, there is no obvious cause; there appears to be no bleeding; no evidence of decreased production or increased destruction of the red blood cells. These are very unsatisfying situations for hematologists because we are so convinced that we should know the cause of the anemia in almost all cases. At the very least, we should know the mechanism of the anemia from the tests we have done: does the patient have decreased production of red cells? Increased red cell destruction? Or is the patient bleeding?

In rare cases in which no cause of anemia is obvious, one hears hoofbeats fine, but instead of thinking about horses, one must think about zebras. I have had two such cases in my career, and they were both truly fascinating. The first patient of this type that I encountered was a young Italian woman who was hospitalized at Hammersmith Hospital in London in 1970 while I was a visiting fellow. I was doing laboratory research there, but I also attended rounds on the service of Sir John Dacie, a noted English physician and hematologist. The young woman patient had a history of a persistent anemia for many years in Italy with no diagnosis, and was referred to Dr. Dacie's world-renowned service for diagnosis and treatment. She was incapacitated by her disease. She was thin, pale, weak, and bed-bound. She needed blood transfusions to maintain her hemoglobin at a reasonable level.

She had had an extensive work-up many times that included all known blood tests and multiple bone marrow examinations in the search for a cause of her anemia. She had no evidence of bleeding or hemolytic anemia, but she did have an increase in the number of so-called "reticulocytes" in her blood. These reticulocytes are young red blood cells that are increased in number in the circulating blood when there is an increased demand for red blood cell production by the marrow, as in patients with either hemolytic anemia or bleeding.

This young woman had increased numbers of reticulocytes, but she had no evidence of either a hemolytic anemia or bleeding. As I have said earlier, the presence of antibodies is evidence of hemolysis. This woman had no such antibodies. Increased red blood cell destruction also leaves behind other laboratory evidence of hemolysis with an increase in the degradation products from increased hemoglobin destruction appearing in blood and urine testing. This patient had negative results of these tests.

So our patient had no diagnosis for a long time. It was the ultimate mystery. She had been hospitalized and closely observed and evaluated in two countries without an explanation for her illness. Then suddenly, someone, not me, made the diagnosis. The patient was discovered to be bleeding herself surreptitiously by inserting a needle into her nose while in the bathroom and letting her blood run into the toilet. She was secretly bleeding herself from a difficult to discover source. The patient had the diagnosis of so-called Munchhausen's syndrome. This is a relatively rare but well-recognized psychiatric illness that remains poorly understood in which patients command medical attention by self-inflicted procedures such as the one this young woman used.

More than two decades passed before I diagnosed a Munchhausen's case of anemia on my own at PH. This time, I was called by a private physician to see his patient, a middle-aged woman. I was rarely consulted by private physicians so I thought this prominent private practitioner had probably approached every other hematologist at PH without success in determining the cause of his patient's anemia when he finally got around to asking me to see her.

The patient was a nurse who had been intensively evaluated with blood and bone marrow tests. She, like the Italian patient I had seen in London so many years before, had an increased reticulocyte count, but no evidence of hemolysis and no source of blood loss. She was debilitated by her illness. She was distraught. She had many blood transfusions that transiently raised her blood count, but then the anemia returned, often quickly.

In this case, antibody blood testing, actually done at another hospital by an expert lab, suggested that an antibody was present in her blood, but it was a minor one, and she had negative results for other tests for the presence of hemolysis. This case was reminiscent to me of my experience with the young woman in England.

Finally, it was decided to more closely observe all of the activities of the patient in her private room. In this case, again, the bathroom was the locale for surreptitious bleeding. The nurse was discovered one day to have inserted a needle into an arm vein from which the blood poured directly into the toilet. The diagnosis was made.

Hematology conferences

As I have said earlier, Thursday was hematology day at CPMC while I was head of hematology and it still is (as of 2012). All of the conferences were held in a conference room on 5 Hudson North on the 5th floor of Milstein Hospital. The room had a long rectangular table around which we hematologists all sat, with guests occupying chairs arrayed along the walls. We spent one hour every Thursday morning from 9–10 AM discussing new patients and follow-ups of previously presented patients with "malignant" hematology: leukemias, lymphomas, myeloma. From 10–11 AM, we discussed hematology patients without cancer, with so-called "non-malignant" or "benign" hematology. Both the full-time academic hematologists (mostly just me) and the practicing hematologists in the division attended along with all of the hematology-oncology fellows and any other physicians or students who wanted to attend, usually 10-20 people. Of all my clinical activities, I was most proud of the quality of these conferences because of the depth of the discussion about the patients and their illnesses.

There were several knowledgeable clinical hematologists consistently around the table. Dr. Gregory Mears, my favorite hematologist, led the discussions of patients with hematological malignancies. Greg had earlier in his career been a hematology-oncology fellow in our program. He had worked in my laboratory for two years, doing research on understanding the genetic basis of thalassemia. He had then gone to Albert Einstein Medical Center to set up his own laboratory and worked there on the genetic aspects of sickle cell disease, investigating why some patients with sickle cell disease were sicker than others. I had recruited him back to Columbia to head the clinical hematology program in the late '80s and appointed him the clinical chief of hematology when he returned. He is still the top clinical hematologist at CPMC today.

The other consistent contributors to these conferences were (and still are): Dr. David Diuguid who, as I have previously mentioned, was the head of the section on coagulation, and who dominated the discussion of coagulation cases; Dr. Michael Flamm, an expert in sickle cell disease and head of the sickle cell program at the Allen Pavilion, an affiliate of CPMC; Dr. David Savage, the leader of bone marrow transplantation at CPMC, and an all-around outstanding clinical hematologist and teacher with major clinical responsibilities at Harlem Hospital; and, for several years, Dr. Bob Reiss, an expert in blood banking and immunologically-based hematologic disorders. Dr. Alice Cohen, an outstanding coagulation expert, and Dr. Harold Ballard, a highly-respected clinician, were intermittent attendees as were other hematology division attendings.

My major contributions to the Thursday morning hematology conferences were to lead the discussions, and to inject any new research perspectives I had into them. We usually spent the first 10-20 minutes on the most interesting new case. The hematology fellow who was consulting on the wards or a medical student taking the hematology elective presented the case and often led a short discussion of the literature relevant to the case, after which there was an informal and open discussion with multiple opinions expressed. I was both a good cop and bad cop to presenters, students or fellows. I think my three closest clinical colleagues, Drs. Mears, Diuguid and Flamm, thought I was sometimes too hard on the fellows. While I never intended to embarrass a presenter, I would not let sloppy thinking pass unnoticed.

There was never a vote about a specific proposal for care. The attending hematologist on the case was usually present and he or she would make the final decision about the further work-up and treatment of the patient. When the hematology attending on the case was not present, the fellow would relay the essentials of the discussion to the absent attending. Although new ward cases took priority, the private hematologists also presented their interesting or difficult private cases as time permitted.

The Hematologic Malignancies Conference at nine AM was also attended regularly by clinical hematopathologists. They presented the appropriate pathological specimens, slides and pictures of biopsies of lymph nodes and bone marrow, when available on the patients to be discussed, and were extremely valuable participants in the conference. Some of the pathologists who attended were also involved in various research studies of the pathophysiology of hematologic malignancies and provided additional and up-to-date insights into the diseases of the patients under discussion. They were heavily involved in the use of new genetic and immunologic markers to categorize different leukemia and lymphoma sub-types. These studies have contributed greatly to the understanding of the pathophysiology of these diseases over the last three decades, and have also been useful in determining the most effective therapies.

I think most of the fellows and attendings in hematology and pathology enjoyed the hematology conferences because they allowed for open discussion of cases by multiple experts and easy participation in the discussions by all. Drug representatives also regularly attended all hematology conferences. Although I knew that they were there primarily to collar private practitioners and promote their particular medications or products in the minutes before and after conferences, I felt that the faculty and fellows were grown-ups who could handle this activity in this particular setting. The drug reps were never allowed to hawk their wares during any hematology conferences, only privately either before or after the conferences. And they seldom approached me.

Caring for in-patients

The Hematology Consult Service was responsible for consulting on all patients with hematologic conditions at PH that we were asked to see by the house staff.

The hematology consult team always consisted of at least one clinical hematology fellow and the attending hematologist. The team was sometimes accompanied by medical students and/or house officers who were taking a hematology elective, and usually made rounds three times a week. The patients' cases were presented in hallways or alcoves, usually by the fellow. Only rarely was a free conference room available to us. On these rounds, the presentations were relatively short as compared to those on ward service rounds, and were focused on the hematology issues. We then always went to the patient's bedside and when I attended I talked to and examined every patient, although doing only a pertinent physical exam. The "hematologist's physical" included a search for jaundice or pallor in the eyes, and for the presence of abnormal lymph nodes and for an enlarged liver and spleen. After our bedside visit, we then discussed the case again. We would then always try to connect with the house officer in charge of the case to update the status of the patient and to discuss the case. We would also review the patient's blood smear, laboratory findings and bone marrow aspirate, if available.

The team would leave a hematology consult note in the patient's chart, at least a preliminary one, within 24 hours of the consult request, and a more detailed one later, summarizing our conclusions. If the consult was an emergency or occurred on days the consult team was not scheduled to go on rounds, the fellow could always beep (or in my case, phone) the attending and arrange to make rounds at the earliest time available.

Most of the patients were on the general medical wards, but those with hematological malignancies were on the "Oncology Ward," first located on the fourth floor of the old Presbyterian Hospital and more recently on a special floor and ward in Millstein Hospital. Daily in-patient rounds on the Oncology Ward were made by an attending team on the ward, usually a hematologist, an oncologist and the house staff; additionally, the Hematology Consult Service consulted on patients with hematologic malignancies on this ward. This dual arrangement allowed for both the in-patient ward team and the hematology clinical fellow and his or her team to be exposed to these very interesting patients. Final decisions about the care of individual in-patients were always in the hands of the in-patient ward team or the private physician, if the patient was a private patient. This was true of all patients at CPMC that I saw or knew about; the final decisions were never in the hands of consults. We as consultants were just that, consultants.

Patients with hematological problems on any of the non-medical wards of the hospital, surgery, ob-gyn, psychiatry, anywhere, were also seen by the hematology consult service. We were rarely consulted on private hematology patients, but we had plenty of business, easily between 30 and 50 new consults each month.

Hematology is not a subspecialty where there are large numbers of patients with emergencies. It is unlike cardiology or gastroenterology where acute heart attacks or bleeding ulcers, respectively, are common and require emergency care. But when there are hematological emergencies, they require prompt and appropriate attention. Hematology attendings were available 24/7 for emergencies, and I remember coming in many times on weekends. This was especially likely with the admission of new patients suspected of having acute leukemia or other life-threatening illnesses such as severe thrombocytopenia (decreased platelets) with bleeding.

The hematology attending was called in all cases that might be diagnosed as acute leukemia. Most often, these cases were straightforward to diagnose and were treated promptly with the institution of special support and chemotherapy. Sometimes, however, the leukemia cases were uncharacteristic and difficult to diagnose. I remember one time in which the fellow called me on a weekend because a patient had severe anemia and thrombocytopenia, signs consistent with a diagnosis of leukemia. He had done a bone marrow examination and had concluded that the patient had acute leukemia with characteristic so-called "blast cells:" in this case, a population of similar monotonous-looking (unvarying and uniform), primitive immature cells present throughout the marrow. When I looked at the marrow I also saw the population of monotonous-looking immature cells, but I knew from my experience that they were not leukemic white blood cells; instead, they were relatively benign cells, so-called "megaloblasts," abnormal red blood cell precursors with specific morphologic diagnostic features caused by vitamin B12 or folic acid deficiency that I had seen many times before but the fellow had not. In fact, the patient had a megaloblastic anemia, a curable anemia.

I was very happy I had been called before the patient was labeled with acute leukemia and treated as such with toxic and unnecessary chemotherapy. The treatment the patient needed in this case was either folic acid or vitamin B12, both given together initially until a specific diagnosis of which deficiency was responsible was made by further testing. Cases of megaloblastic anemia mistakenly first diagnosed as acute leukemia have been reported in the literature only rarely, but probably occur more often.

Another interesting case that I recall to this day is that of a middle aged man, Mr. K., who had acute promyelocytic leukemia (APL). APL is a treatable, even potentially curable form of acute leukemia. The malignant cells are more mature than the immature primitive-looking blast cells seen in other forms of acute leukemia. Mr. K. was treated with appropriate chemotherapy as well as retinoic acid, the latter a unique therapy that helps eliminate the abnormal APL cells. His APL cells disappeared, but during the course of his hospitalization and treatment, Mr. K. developed kidney failure and went into a coma, presumably because of the chemotherapy he received. The problem in this patient was not strictly a hematological or medical issue, but a social one. Neither Mr. K. nor any of his relatives had agreed to a "do not resuscitate" (DNR) order. Without such an order, we were doing all we could as the medical and hematology team, along with the intensive care unit team, to keep Mr. K. alive, including renal dialysis until his renal function improved and until the toxic effects of his chemotherapy wore off. At issue was what Mr. K.'s own wishes would most likely have been if he were conscious and able to make his own judgment about his continued care. A further complication of the case was that it was unclear who was his responsible next of kin: a woman he lived with, or a cousin of his, his closest living relative.

Mr. K.'s leukemia was in remission (there were no APL cells), yet he was in a coma. I always feel that in this type of situation, in which chemotherapy had helped the patient improve and there is a reasonable expectation of recovery, we physicians should pull out all the stops and do our utmost. We are able to support patients in coma effectively, although with great effort, and often in these cases the results are favorable if the underlying condition improves with treatment, as seemed to be the case with Mr. K.'s leukemia.

After several meetings that included Mr. K.'s relatives and the woman he lived with and the intensive care unit staff and we hematologists, we decided to continue to support him intensively and continue his renal dialysis despite his coma. Happily, Mr. K. finally awoke, improved rapidly and went home. When he recovered and I talked with him about his views on his treatment while he was in a coma, of course he was happy with our decisions; it was clear that he was glad to be alive and to be able to go home.

I also remember the end of Mr. K.'s story. We were elated about Mr. K.'s recovery, and the fellow proudly reported the details of our success on Thursday morning rounds. While everyone was upbeat, Dr. Mears warned us not to be too happy: that the remission might be only temporary. Sadly, Dr. Mears was right, and Mr. K. relapsed a few months later, did not respond to further therapy, and died. Our treatment had not cured Mr. K., but I wouldn't have done anything different if I had it all to do over again.

I believe that my status as an academic physician with only limited clinical responsibilities allowed me to be more emotionally involved in the care of patients like Mr. K. than many other physicians, especially full time-clinicians. Full-time clinicians are constantly confronted with highly charged emotional situations like Mr. K.'s in which patients are critically ill and in which proper and intense treatment will largely determine the outcome. This is a tremendous responsibility and takes an enormous emotional toll that eventually leads to a controlled turning down of the emotional volume by these physicians, as it must for their continued sanity.

I, on the other hand, only had to worry about patient care problems for relatively limited periods of time. I could afford to have more highs and lows in response to success or failure in the care of individual patients. Also, having highs and lows was part of my personality. Cases like Mr. K.'s engulfed me in terms of feelings as well as thinking, much more so than any laboratory experiment did. Success, when it occurred in the care of a patient like Mr. K., was as thrilling to me as any exhilaration that I felt when I discovered something new in the laboratory. It was the thrill of helping a fellow human in serious distress. Being a scientist, you enjoy the process of doing experiments and revel in the occasional positive result. As a clinician, every result in every patient counts.

Overall, I thought our care of ward patients with hematological problems at CPMC was superb.

CHAPTER THIRTEEN

Sickle Cell Disease

While my life in the laboratory was focused on the genetic defects in thalassemia, an inherited anemia, my clinical activities were largely focused on the care of patients with another inherited disorder of hemoglobin, sickle cell disease. Thalassemia is primarily a disease of children and is managed primarily by pediatric hematologists even after the children grow into adulthood. Many more adult patients with sickle cell disease than with thalassemia are cared for by adult hematologists like me. CPMC was a major center for the care of patients with sickle cell disease during my entire tenure and remains so today. Their clinical care is difficult and demanding for physicians since they are both chronically ill and have many acute medical problems.

The disease is called "sickle cell" because the patients' red blood cells become deformed into the shape of curved, slender sickles when low oxygen is present; the sickling is due to the presence in the patients' red blood cells of an abnormal hemoglobin, sickle cell hemoglobin; the abnormal hemoglobin is the result of a small change in the DNA of these patients who are mainly of African descent. The anemia is due to the fact that the sickled red blood cells are destroyed prematurely. Normally, red blood cells live for over 100 days in our circulation; sickle red cells live less than a tenth as long.

The most common and nagging problem in patients with sickle cell disease is sickle cell "painful crises," in which the sickled red blood cells clog small blood vessels, leading to ischemia (lack of oxygen) of the tissues and pain. This ischemia and pain is analogous to what occurs in patients with coronary artery disease when their heart muscle does not get enough oxygen due to reduced blood flow.

Painful crises are heart-wrenching experiences for sickle patients. Uncontrollable, unpredictable bouts of sudden severe disabling pain can occur most anywhere, but primarily in the arms, legs, abdomen and chest, and come without warning to overwhelm the patient. They feel paralyzed by the pain. The pain drives the patients to despair, and they are totally dependent on their physicians for pain control and support during these traumatic episodes. Because of the frequent occurrence of these severe painful episodes, the bond between doctor and patient in sickle cell disease is extremely important. While every patient needs one primary physician to care for them, this need is never more urgent than for these patients. They especially need care by a doctor who trusts them because sickle cell painful crisis is most often unaccompanied by objective physical signs or by blood tests that make a definitive diagnosis. The physician caring for the patient has to rely on the patient's history of the subjective feeling of pain. The doctor must trust the patient's story and judgment. If the doctor knows the patient well, there is usually no problem.

However, if the patient appears for the first time in an emergency room or in a doctor's office where he or she is not known, there are often problems, particularly since many sickle patients in painful crisis demand and require large amounts of narcotics for pain relief. Physicians unfamiliar with the care of these patients may surmise that the patients are simply drug addicts, feigning their pain and using it as an excuse to receive narcotics.

Although most sickle cell patients are drug dependent, in fact, only rarely are they truly addicted. They come to the hospital only when their pain is so severe that they need parenteral (non-oral) medication. They need medication to treat their pain, not primarily because of their psychological or physical craving for drugs. Sickle cell patients rely on their doctors for their pain medication when they need it. They cannot afford to be disbelieved and rebuffed by their physicians. They need their doctor's trust.

Sickle cell anemia patients also understand that they will sometimes require high levels of narcotics to control their pain when they have a severe crisis. Therefore, the patients cannot afford to become tolerant to high doses of narcotics because then they will be less responsive to these medications at a time when they most need their pain-relieving effects.

The psychosocial problems of sickle cell patients further complicate their care. Most of the patients are poor or middle class and largely unemployed. Their chronic illness and frequent hospitalizations make it difficult for them to hold jobs, even when, during the periods that their disease is under control, they are able and willing to do so. The government-sponsored Medicaid program has been a godsend for these chronically ill patients, and is critical in allowing them to receive the care they need.

Caring

I am particularly proud of the way we treated sickle cell patients at Columbia-Presbyterian during my many years there. We continuously followed between 150 and 200 adults with the disease at CPMC and treated them with sensitivity and respect. We gave them as much pain medicine as they needed to control their pain. Although most sickle cell patients are quite manageable primarily as outpatients in hematology clinic, there were a few who were more seriously ill and/or were truly addicted to the pain medication who were seen in the Emergency Room, sometimes several times a week demanding medication; some of these patients also went to other hospital emergency rooms as well with the same demands for pain relief.

If a sickle cell patient came to our CPMC emergency room and had severe enough pain requiring admission, that was done. If the pain or other medical problem was not severe enough for admission, the patient was sent home, but with only enough potent narcotic pills like dilaudid or oxycontin to treat the pain until the next hematology clinic visit, usually the next Tuesday afternoon.

Most patients relied on acetaminophen (Tylenol) and codeine to treat mild painful crises at home. When these drugs failed, the patients often had a few oral dilaudid or oxycontin pills on hand to try to ride out the crisis for a few days before either coming to the clinic or the emergency room, despite the risk that some patients would become dependent on these oral medications. A few patients were on oral morphine. I never liked using oral morphine as outpatient medication. We reserved parenteral (non-oral) medications for severe painful crisis requiring hospital admission. When patients were admitted with severe crisis, they were treated with either meperidine (Demerol) or morphine given by injection. Morphine given intravenously by patient-controlled administration (PCA) is often used to treat painful crises today. PCA, in which the patient controls the amount of morphine received, within limits, has been found to be a most effective way to treat hospitalized patients with sickle cell painful crises.

As with other patients, we tried to have a specific hematologist follow each sickle cell patient regularly in hematology clinic. This system of having a specific primary doctor for each patient, whether it was a fellow, resident or attending physician, was a general policy at PH, and, as I have said before, is critical for optimal patient care.

We had what I consider an extraordinary group of hematology attending physicians taking care of our sickle cell patients as well as all other hematology patients from the '80s until I left in 2005 (all are still there today). They included many of the same doctors I have mentioned earlier: Drs. Mears, Diuguid, Flamm, Savage and I were the core group who also supervised the care given by residents and fellows to sickle cell patients. I will always think of these colleagues as the best group of doctors I ever worked with. It surprises me now to recall that we, as a group, spent over 20 years working together — making rounds, having conferences, seeing patients and teaching house staff and fellows at Columbia-Presbyterian. The time passed so smoothly with very few unpleasant experiences, at least for me, and was marked by high quality care, companionship and professional camaraderie. These physicians were all mainly in some level of private practice except for me, but they were also dedicated to teaching and to an academic approach to the best care of patients. Although they were all extremely busy with practice, they always had time for academic pursuits, such as conferences, rounds, and mentoring.

Our hematology division had an advantage over programs at other hospitals in taking care of sickle cell patients since all of us, Mears, Diuguid, Flamm, Savage and I, were all experts on sickle cell disease. Savage had trained at Harlem Hospital with Dr. John Lindenbaum, another sickle cell expert, and saw many sickle cell patients there. As I have said, Mears had worked with sickle cell patients during his academic career at Albert Einstein and at CPMC, and Flamm was a fellow in our program particularly interested in caring for patients with this disease. David Diuguid, who primarily saw patients with clotting and bleeding disorders, also had extensive experience caring for sickle cell disease patients. All of us taking care of sickle cell patients were on the same page. To some degree, we were all true academic so-called "triple-threats:" we had done research; we knew clinical medicine; and we were good teachers.

Our adult hematology group at CPMC participated in many national programs involving sickle cell disease. For much of the '70s to the'90s we had a Comprehensive Sickle Cell Center, one of relatively few funded by the NIH, with a variety of sickle cell projects, including antenatal diagnosis of the disease; newborn screening; research into the rheological changes (changes in the flow characteristics) of sickle cells; and studies of potential new treatments for the disease, including gene therapy. Along with the adult patients, there were also 150–200 children with sickle disease followed by pediatric hematologists at Children's Hospital at CPMC. Dr. Sergio Piomelli, a scientist and pediatrician, led the Sickle Cell Center for many years. Drs. Jeanne Smith and Doris Wethers, at Harlem Hospital and St. Luke's-Roosevelt, respectively, also contributed to the Center's activities.

A complex disease

There is tremendous variability in the clinical manifestations of different patients with sickle cell disease. Although all of the patients inherit the same two sickle cell genes, some patients are seen frequently for painful crises and other problems and require intensive care, while others are relatively well. Obviously, other genetic and environmental factors account for this variability. The search for these factors has been ongoing for decades. High on the list of candidates to account for this clinical variability is the role of fetal hemoglobin, the predominant hemoglobin found primarily in fetal life. Sickle cell patients with higher levels of fetal hemoglobin have less severe disease manifestations than those with lower fetal hemoglobin levels. In the last two decades, a drug, hydroxyurea, has been found to increase fetal hemoglobin levels to a limited extent which, together with the drug's other beneficial effects, diminishes the number of sickle cell painful crises in both adult patients and children with the disease.

Sickle cell anemia is a multisystem disease, and patients have many complications other than sickle cell painful crises. The anemia in sickle cell disease is a so-called "well-compensated" hemolytic anemia in which vastly increased production of red cells produced in the bone marrow of these patients compensates for the increased destruction (hemolysis) of the sickle blood cells in the circulating blood. As long as these patients do not have conditions that restrict their capacity for increased red blood cell production, most of them do not need blood transfusions. However, when red blood cell production by the bone marrow is curtailed for any reason, severe anemia can ensue. Folic acid deficiency and infections are the most common reasons for this occurrence. Normally, sickle cell patients are routinely treated with oral folic acid supplements to prevent deficiency. When severe anemia occurs in patients with sickle cell disease, they are, of course, given blood transfusions.

Despite relatively well-tolerated modest anemia in most patients, chronic damage to the lungs, heart, liver, and bones almost always eventually occurs as the result of the anemia and of sickling. Sickling in certain areas of the body which normally have a limited blood supply, such as the shoulders and hips, often leads to so-called "aseptic necrosis," bone damage and death of bone in these areas. These complications often require surgical replacement of these joints. Limited blood flow to the retina of the eye can cause decreased vision and blindness in these patients.

Distortions of blood flow in cerebral blood vessels due to sickled cells is a common and serious complication in sickle cell disease that can lead to recurrent strokes and seizures and death, especially in children. Multiple controlled clinical trials have shown that blood transfusions can prevent these complications. The need for continued long-term transfusions to prevent recurrent strokes in these patients has been documented.

Transfusions in sickle cell disease are usually given by "exchange transfusion"; in this procedure, the patient's sickle cell blood is removed by vein and the patient is transfused with (given), also by vein, intravenously (IV), non-sickle blood in exchange. The idea behind this therapy is to dilute the sickle red blood cells by adding enough normal red blood cells to prevent the sickling of the blood and its complications. In the '60s to '80s, I and others like me performed exchange transfusion manually by sticking a needle into the vein of a patient at the bedside, removing a unit of blood, and then giving one or more units of non-sickle blood to the patient by transfusion, and sometimes repeating this procedure. In the last several decades, this manual procedure has rarely been used because of the availability of so-called "apheresis" machines which, using two IVs, mechanically and automatically allow the exchange to be done, with the patient's cells removed and normal cells transfused simultaneously. Exchange transfusion is often used rather than simply the transfusion of normal blood alone since the exchange process more rapidly increases the percent of normal cells relative to sickle cells, and it limits the total amount of blood the patient accumulates.

A major complication of frequent blood transfusions, including exchange transfusions, is that they can lead to excessive iron deposition, especially in the heart, and to heart failure and death due to the presence of iron in the hemoglobin of the transfused red blood cells. Until the '90s, the only effective method for removing iron, iron chelation therapy, was by the laborious use of desferioxamine (Desferal), given subcutaneously by pump for 10–12 hours nightly five times a week. This was unacceptable treatment for most sickle cell patients. Today, effective oral iron chelators are available for this purpose, and are being used more extensively in patients who need to be chronically transfused.

Patients with sickle cell disease can also have immunological problems and can develop bacterial pneumonias. Pneumococcal pneumonia previously killed many children with the disease, but today they are routinely given pneumococcal vaccine in early life to prevent this dangerous complication. A "chest syndrome," due to either pneumonia or to small or large blood clots (pulmonary thrombosis), can also occur in these patients. Relatively recently, another type of lung problem caused by sickling, pulmonary hypertension, has been recognized. In this condition, increased pressure in the major blood vessels in the lungs can lead to sudden heart failure and death. Many centers now use exchange transfusions to treat chest syndrome and pulmonary hypertension, although the effectiveness of this treatment has not been shown in controlled clinical trials. There is no strong evidence that routine use of exchange transfusions modifies the history of painful crises in most patients although it is sometimes used and found to be beneficial in some patients with severe recurrent crises.

The treatment of sickle cell disease is a great challenge for doctors and patients. It is a chronic disease that can be managed, but it requires extraordinary and persistent medical care. Although patients with sickle disease have reduced life expectancy, many patients live into their 40s and 50s and some beyond. I remember most of the relatively few sickle cell patients who died on my watch. I was always very surprised and upset when they died because I believed that we should have been able to effectively treat all of these patients' sickle cell complications. I remember one patient who routinely received Demerol, one of the drugs used to treat severe painful crises but that can also cause seizures. Despite our best efforts, she died of uncontrolled seizures and aspiration pneumonia. Another patient died because of an uncontrolled pneumonia and an accompanying pericardial effusion. There were also rare sickle cell patients who died because of unrecognized rapidly progressing anemia.

As has been shown in several clinical trials, continuing to treat sickle cell patients with previous strokes and seizures with blood transfusions has been proven to be effective in preventing new cerebrovascular events. I remember one young patient who died of these complications. He was a Jehovah's witness and his family refused on religious grounds to have him continue to be treated with blood transfusions. I was very frustrated about this case, but my colleagues and I could not convince the family to allow us to continue to give him blood transfusions, despite the dire medical situation of this young patient, since, at the time, we had no strong scientific evidence that continuing blood transfusion support could be life-saving.

Despite the fact that we scientists and physicians have known the cause and pathophysiology of sickle cell disease for over 60 years, it is sad that, at present, we have no cure for the majority of patients. However, some patients can be cured with allogeneic bone marrow transplantation, a procedure through which they receive adequate normal blood stem cells from an HLA-matched sibling or other donor with many of the same immunologic markers as their own. Gene therapy, inserting a normal hemoglobin gene into the patient's own blood stem cells, an approach I worked on in the laboratory for many years, is also a potential cure. This treatment is still in the early stages of clinical development and has not been used in sickle cell patients as yet.

For families at risk for sickle cell disease, in which both parents have sickle cell trait, antenatal (or prenatal) diagnosis is readily available, if sought. Diagnostic testing can be done early in pregnancy by biopsy of chorionic villi (part of the placenta), or later, by amniocentesis, removal of fluid containing fetal cells from the pregnant woman. DNA analysis of the samples leads to rapid and accurate diagnosis. However, the availability of antenatal diagnosis and acceptance of genetic testing in the appropriate ethnic communities are necessary for these programs to be successful. In addition, genetic counseling must also be available for discussion of antenatal diagnosis and of possible subsequent termination of pregnancy. To date, antenatal diagnosis has had only limited effectiveness in reducing the incidence of sickle cell disease.

CHAPTER FOURTEEN

Special People

Gladys

Gladys Jacobs, now 63, is one of the many African-American patients with sickle cell disease that I cared for at PH. Beginning in the 1970s, I was her hematologist when she came to Hematology Clinic and her consulting hematologist when she was admitted to the medical wards at Presbyterian Hospital. Early on, I saw her on the 10th floor of an old clinic building, Vanderbilt Clinic, a part of the old Presbyterian Hospital at 168th Street and Broadway. Later, I cared for her in the newer out-patient clinic facilities in Atchley Pavilion (now Irving Pavilion) across Fort Washington Avenue.

After leaving Columbia, I found out in 2007 that Gladys was living at the Beth Abraham Nursing Home, a chronic nursing facility in the Bronx, and I decided to see her again, this time as a friend and as a possible subject for this book. It was a glorious fall day when I first went to visit her from my home, only 10–15 minutes away by car. The greens and yellows and oranges and browns of the trees filled the avenues and parks along the way as I drove from Riverdale to Moshulu Parkway, past the Botanical Gardens, and entered the street of the nursing facility, Allerton Avenue, just off the Bronx River Parkway. Since that first visit, I have seen Gladys several more times.

There was a stark contrast between the beauty of the outdoors scene I had passed on my trip and the inside of Beth Abraham with its gray caravans of wheelchairs, many carrying patients, clogging the halls. It was clean inside, the floors newly waxed, almost sterile-looking. Gladys was in a semi-private room on the 7th floor of the facility, part of a modified hospital ward with a corridor filled with private and semi-private hospital rooms reminiscent to me of the old Presbyterian Hospital. She had one small closet in the room for all her clothes, and a small dresser for all of her other personal belongings.

On that first visit, I sit in the one chair near her bed to talk to her. The other occupant of the room is fortunately absent. Only a thin cloth partition separates the two patient bed areas. Gladys is doing a word puzzle with fill-ins. She gives me a warm wide smile and seems happy to see me. When she was my patient in the old days, she was usually quite reserved and unemotional. She seems more relaxed with me now. Gladys is physically and mentally much as I remember her when she was my patient. She has always been a very rational person, even under stress; her emotions are almost always under tight control; her voice is usually strong, and her complaints usually justified. She smiles more now than she ever did as a patient of mine in the old days.

"We butted heads a few times, but you were OK," Gladys tells me in that first meeting more than 30 years after I first saw her. "Everyone at Columbia-Presbyterian treated me well. With respect." She reminds me that she didn't like it when, as a young physician, I lumped her with other sickle cell patients, "I'm Gladys, I told you. I'm not just another sickler." But aside from my disrespecting her in this way, she was happy with my care. "You cared. Most of the doctors at Presbyterian really cared." I am happy to hear her say that we had treated her well back then, and I tell her so. She tells me that the only hospital she really trusts for care is Columbia-Presbyterian. She does not like being treated at other hospitals. "If the ambulance ever tried to take me to another hospital, I'd scream my head off."

She is now under the care of Dr. Delfine Taylor, a physician in general medicine at PH. She thinks that having a doctor in general medicine like Dr. Taylor is better than having a hematologist as her primary physician because she feels that Dr. Taylor is more accessible than hematologists like me were and are more readily available to take care of her multiple medical problems.

Towards the end of the first visit with her, I help Gladys with her wheelchair, and she takes me to her favorite spot, the backyard or courtyard of the building that, in fair weather, is filled with other patients in wheelchairs. It is an outdoor refuge, away from the tight quarters and confinement of the hospital in-patient facility. And she can smoke there. It has a large flat concrete surface, unadorned. There is no colorful view of the beautiful trees and grass outside nearby. All that can be seen from the backyard are the tops of brick buildings visible over the fence.

Gladys tells me on that first visit, and subsequently, that she feels trapped. Because of sickle cell disease affecting her hip joints, she cannot walk without support; she has hip pain and limitation of motion due to hip replacements. "The left one keeps slippin' out, many times." She needs a wheelchair to get around, and has recently received a motorized one that makes her mobility considerably greater. She also has had shoulder surgery, again for problems secondary to her disease. "I couldn't get around with a regular wheelchair without someone pushing it because one of my shoulders didn't work after my shoulder replacement a while ago.

"Finally, one day, the motorized wheelchair appeared at my door. For the last six months I've tried to get permission to use it to go outside of the hospital and enjoy the neighborhood. The therapy department has to give me a test for me to do that. They haven't got around to it yet even though I have used the chair for months now. It just takes forever to get anything done around here."

By now, Gladys has been in Beth Abraham for over six years, much longer than she ever thought she would be. She had developed an infection of her left shoulder after surgery at PH, and since there was no one to care for her at home when she was ready to be discharged, she was sent to Beth Abraham instead. Her old apartment was lost to her along the way." It was supposed to be 'temporary.' Can you imagine, six years here and the social workers can't find me nothin', now that I want to be by myself. I don't think they want me to leave. I think they like me staying here. I have no privacy here." Things have gotten a bit better for her at Beth Abraham recently. She has been moved into a corner single room on the seventh floor that is quite an upgrade from her old room, and she now has her own bathroom and privacy. She has applied for an apartment nearby the Beth Abraham Home but has been disappointed several times. Recently (October 2011), she was close to obtaining an apartment but so far, no luck. She will require a home health aide if she does move.

Gladys has few visitors. Her sister, two years older than her, lives in Co-op City, a few miles away, only 15 minutes by car. "I have a family from outer space," she tells me during my first visit, "Can you imagine?

She's visited me six times in two years, and when she does she barely has time to sit down. She's supposed to be working with the social worker and my doctor to find me an apartment, but she hasn't done a thing. My family is no help at all. And the staff here does only what is necessary." In my opinion, the Beth Abraham facility is not all bad for Gladys: she now has the private room; it is a clean place; there is adequate nursing and custodial personnel; it has a library. Gladys reads books, plays bingo and does her fill-in word puzzles in her spare time. She smokes her Marlboro 100 cigarettes in the backyard as often as she can and lounges there often when the weather permits.

Gladys was one of the first sickle cell patients I saw in the hematology clinic and wards of Presbyterian Hospital. Her clinical disease was somewhat milder than some other patients, but she certainly has had many painful crises and extensive bone involvement as a result of her disease. She has had a long hard life. She lived in Harlem as a child with her single mother who had drug and alcohol problems. She is one of nine siblings. According to Gladys, she was rejected by her mother and was sent intermittently to be raised in foster homes when younger siblings came along, only to be returned to her biological mother's care on occasion.

She went to a Catholic elementary school and was graduated from George Washington High School. She worked full-time for many years, from her teens into her 30s, as a file clerk in a federal civil service job in the immigration service at 20 West Broadway and later at 26 Federal Plaza. She loved the job and was happy in the workplace. She was moving up the civil service ladder. However, because of her frequent absences due to her hospitalizations for sickle cell painful crises, she eventually had to revert to part-time work. She was finally forced to either resign or be laid off. She resigned.

The loss of her job was a terrible blow to her ego and her life. She could never again find a stable job after that, was supported by disability benefits and Medicaid, and was forced to stay in a small apartment in Harlem. "Once I stopped working, it took my whole world away from me." She became depressed and was in Psychiatric Institute for long periods, including when I saw her as a hematology patient. When she was out of the hospital, she lived with other females in an apartment in Washington Heights.

She became pregnant by her fiance when she was in her twenties, but lost the baby six weeks into the pregnancy. Soon after that, she found out that her fiance had drowned in an accident in a Brooklyn pool.

Gladys has taken extensive pain medication over the years for her painful crises and for her chronic hip and shoulder pains. She has gone through the gamut of oral medications: Tylenol, codeine, and Dilaudid and is currently dependent on oral morphine. When she has severe painful crises and is admitted to PH, she uses patient-controlled administration (PCA) of intravenous morphine. She used to be treated by me and other physicians with intramuscular Demerol, but, she says, "it's very painful and leads to knots in my body. I don't like it. The PCA morphine is much better." She also says, "There are some sickle patients who use the medication just to get high. I only use it for pain." I believe her. That to me is the difference between drug addiction and drug dependence. Gladys only uses the parenteral narcotics for pain.

At the request of Dr. Taylor, Gladys agrees to be seen by and to talk to the first year class at the College of Physicians and Surgeons, Columbia University's medical school, as part of a course introducing young students to patients. She likes the experience; she doesn't mind the exposure and doesn't feel exploited. She feels she is "giving back something" for the extensive care she has received at Columbia-Presbyterian. Since I first visited her at Beth Abraham, Gladys has had several sickle cell painful crises and a neurological event, "either a small stroke or a seizure, doctors aren't sure," from which she has recovered.

Gladys has been excited recently (2012) because she has finally gotten to the top of the list of patients who are eligible to be transferred from the nursing facility to their own apartments, outside the hospital, but nearby. Having listened to Gladys complain of her troubles getting on this list for years now, I am happy for her, although I can't help being concerned about her living alone now at the age of 63, even with the supportive services of a home health aide. She is barely able to walk because of her bilateral hip replacements, one of which has been continually troublesome. But I am rooting for her, and she is rooting hard for herself. I am happy that she still feels hope and optimism for the future. So I support her hopes for a day when she can finally be on her own, move into her own private living space, and feel independent and free again for as long as possible.

Vinnie

While Gladys is trapped in the web of Medicaid and public housing and medical facilities, Vinnie Vitale, a special friend of mine over recent decades, was not. Vinnie was a former New York State judge who had all the medical care he needed all his life. When he retired, he had good medical insurance with Medicare and supplemental coverage. Montefiore Hospital was the central hub of his care. He had major cardiac surgery there, and received continuous care by Montefiore doctors, including during recent hospitalizations for carotid artery obstruction and abnormal heart rhythms.

Vinnie lived in an apartment building in Riverdale which houses medical offices that included the office of his internist, essentially his family doctor. In contrast to Gladys, he always had immediate access to all the services he needed: ambulances, home health care, emergency care.

The last Wednesday in July 2010, we played poker, as usual, in the dining area off his living room, and he was his usual happy self. Seymour, Barry, Ralph, Craig, and I were the other players. Six or seven make a good poker game. We had had our usual pizza break at 9:30 and Vinnie enjoyed his slice.

We had resumed playing and when it was his turn to ante his quarter, he turned to me and said, "I can't move my hand." I asked if he was OK and he said, "No. I don't feel well." With that, he needed support to sit up. I wanted him to lie down to get the blood going to his head, but I couldn't move him. He weighs over 200 pounds. Barry who weighs about as much as Vinnie and is the only youngster in the game (he's in his 40s), right then and there, with a deep breath and a bear hug that I will never forget, lifted Vinnie up and set him down flat on his back on the couch in the living room. I don't know what we all would have done with Vinnie without Barry's help, probably we would have simply tried to slide Vinnie gently from the chair to the floor.

With Vinnie on the couch, I checked his pulse, which was regular, strong and steady, and asked him if he could move his arms and legs. He said he could but then he and I noticed that his right leg was weak. He could barely move it. Then he began slurring his speech. We called 911.

We began clearing the poker table and Vinnie asked how much money he had. When told, he said, "I lost five dollars." I asked him how he was feeling, and he said, "I think I'm having a stroke." It was the last thing I remember him saying.

Two EMS people came in 15 minutes, checked him, and took him to the Allen Pavilion despite our firm request that they take him to Montefiore where he was a known patient. At the Allen, he was unconscious and found to have a cerebral hemorrhage. The doctors there reversed the anticoagulation he was on (which could have contributed to his bleeding), and transferred him to the ICU at Milstein Hospital at Columbia-Presbyterian for further care. Barry went with him, and reported his progress to me over the next couple of days. He never regained consciousness. By Sunday, I heard he was made DNR (do not rescusitate) and DNI (do not intubate). I felt I had to see him alive one more time that day.

I drove down to PH and went to his room. He was unconscious and unresponsive, even to deep pain stimuli. He seemed comfortable and at peace and was breathing shallowly. His room had a beautiful view of the Hudson River, but he could not enjoy it. I talked to him about the poker game and how we all hoped he would feel better even though I knew he did not, in all probability, hear me. I stayed for a while watching him. I talked to a nurse who knew his condition, and she told me he was not doing well. She wouldn't let me see his chart since I was no longer on the medical staff. I didn't object. I had nothing to add to his care.

I called Barry as I walked to my car that Sunday afternoon on the familiar streets of Washington Heights, and I told him that I had seen Vinnie and that he was not doing well. I was glad I had seen him one last time, more for myself than for Vinnie. Barry called me at 10 PM that night to tell me that Vinnie had died.

We should have had another poker game instead of a wake. As it turned out, we had neither. The funeral was Thursday, August 5th 2010 at 10 AM at St. Gabriel's Church. It was a traditional Catholic service. There were only 20 or so people there in the small church and chapel including several of us from the weekly poker game.

Vinnie was my friend and I loved him. We had many good times together: at the poker table; just sitting around in his apartment; at Dominic's on Arthur Avenue having shrimp and linguini with white clam sauce, and stuffed baked clams. He loved going to Arthur Avenue. He grew up in a neighborhood not far from there, near the Bronx Zoo and the

Botanical Gardens. One night, after an early Dominic's dinner, I drove him past the two houses he had lived in during his youth. He was excited to see that those houses were still intact. I think he really enjoyed that tour.

Vinnie was already frail when I first met him and he had grown more frail over the years. He had had a coronary bypass, hypertension, diabetes, and a stroke, but he still was up and around and working as a judge until a few years ago. And when it came to poker or eating or the Mets or friendship, he never flagged. He was up for anything. Whenever we went out to eat, people would usually recognize him from his days as a judge and come over to our table and introduce themselves and wish him well. He was quite well known in the Bronx, Judge Vincent Vitale.

Vinnie sometimes had a stern look on his face that could put people off, but he also had a wonderfully sincere and gentle smile that those of us who loved him knew so well. He could hardly walk over the last year of his life, but we kept going to Arthur Avenue and playing poker. He also had two cataract operations during the last year of his life. He was reading again and could see his poker cards and his food and his beloved Mets better. Vinnie's death left me with a great sadness.

PART FOUR

Medicine Today

CHAPTER FIFTEEN

The Practice of Medicine

The real world for doctors

Practicing medicine today is much more complicated than it used to be when I was an active physician. This is particularly true in the private practice of medicine. There have been drastic changes over recent decades due to the expanded role of government in medical care as our population ages and becomes poorer and less able to afford private medical insurance, and to the expanded role of large for-profit insurance companies as intermediaries in our medical reimbursement system. However, even as practice conditions in the world of medicine have drastically changed, almost all doctors continue to have their patients' best interests and optimal care as their goal, and are as dedicated to their profession and to their patients as they ever were.

Almost all physicians enter the profession of medicine primarily because they want to take care of patients. I certainly did. Some like me end up doing mostly research and teaching. Others become involved in public health or become medical administrators. Very few physicians enter medicine primarily for its financial rewards. The long road to becoming a physician, typically with many loans along the way, constitutes too arduous a journey to justify if the goal is simply that of making money. However, aspiring doctors know that a career in medicine eventually ensures at the very least a reasonable income, and provides long-term financial security. I know that financial security was at least part of the equation in my mind when I decided to become a doctor.

Sadly, over the past 30 years, medical care in America has become much more of a big business than ever before. As a result of an ever-burgeoning health care-for-profit-of-private-investors industry, we have all, doctors and patients alike, become the victims medically, financially and emotionally of a fragmented health care system. Many of our citizens in the US are uninsured; they receive either no or poor health care. We are the only developed country in the world, other than a few in the former USSR, that does not recognize universal health care as a right rather than a privilege, does not provide health care for all of its citizens, and does not have the costs of care regulated by the government. Physician fees and hospital costs have risen constantly in the United States, and drug and device and testing costs have skyrocketed. Most importantly, companies and corporations, small and large, with their primary focus on maximizing returns for their investors, have changed much of medical care from a professional calling to big business.

For-profit Health Maintenance Organizations (HMOs) are parts of insurance companies that have become more and more dominant in recent decades in the high finance of fee-for-service medicine. These private for-profit managed care organizations have increased in number and influence as well. These mega-businesses have interfered with the traditional relationships between doctors and their patients by their imposition of new intrusive rules for doctors and patients, often requiring pre approval for medical services, if they are to reimburse costs at all, and requiring much more paperwork from physicians than they ever had before. These managed care programs have made it much more difficult for physicians to take care of patients and to afford to do so in traditional ways. Many private doctors who used to earn reasonable incomes 25 years ago have been totally overwhelmed by the changing patterns of medical practice and medical reimbursement over the past two decades, and have stopped participating in these plans.

Overall, the addition of managed care insurance to more traditional private insurance plans and the concomitant development of new patterns of physician and patient care reimbursement has contaminated medical practice, fragmented care and increased costs. Delayed, low and sometimes denied reimbursement for medical services by insurers have made current private medical practice a nightmare for many physicians who have stayed in these insurance programs.

HMOs have the power to control reimbursements to physicians and patients and, by Federal law, cannot be sued for malpractice; only individual doctors can. With these ground rules, many of these insurance providers have felt they have a green light to do all they can to deny reimbursement for care. They have legions of employees, some of whose only job is to find reasons to deny payment to doctors and patients for services, which partially explains why they have huge administrative costs. These costs, which are much greater than those of government programs like Medicare and Medicaid, and those of ordinary private practice or group practices, are met by the ever-increasing premiums that employers and patients' themselves are forced to pay. Although these companies control reimbursement to doctors, hospitals and patients, however, it should be emphasized that drug and device companies as well as hospitals and doctors themselves try to set the highest prices to be charged for their products and services, and are major contributors to the continuing rise of our total health care costs as a nation. In September 2011, it was reported in the New York Times (NYT), one of my many public sources of medical information for this book also including journals, government reports and other media, that the average cost of medical care had risen 9% over the previous year to over $15,000 per family.

There are, of course, some exceptions to this grim picture that might herald reform in the system in the future. Group practices have been established all over the country that are able to more effectively control their costs because they bundle their services and are therefore able to provide patient care at more reasonable fees. Kaiser Permanente and Cleveland Clinic are among the best examples of efficient and available medical care. Excellent devoted doctors deliver excellent, affordable and prompt care. New so-called accountable care organizations (ACOs), groups of physicians that collaborate to provide more integrated care and services, and have lower fees, are springing up as well. But these group practices, some for-profit and some non-profit, represent only a small portion of the total medical care system in the US today.

The federal government is trying its best to meet the medical needs of the poor and the elderly, via Medicaid and Medicare, respectively. These programs have expanded greatly in recent years. However, political pressure to rein in the increasing costs of these services to an aging and sicker population covered by Medicare and to an expanding poorer population covered by Medicaid has led to decreased government reimbursement to physicians and hospitals for the care and treatment of patients in these programs.

Reliable figures on the true incomes of physicians are difficult to come by and confirm. Published estimates of the average net incomes of internists are currently between $150,000 and $250,000 a year. Specialists in internal medicine like cardiologists, gastroenterologists and oncologists, and other specialists like surgeons, urologists, orthopedists, dermatologists, ophthalmologists, radiologists, and anesthesiologists make much more, often over $500,000, and sometimes into the millions. Many physicians are in the top one percent of the nation's earners (NYT). Most of these high-earning physicians provide high quality medical care while commanding their high incomes. Among them are some of the best doctors I know. However, rising medical care costs in the United States are at least partially due to the increasing reimbursements being paid to sustain or increase the incomes of these physicians over the past several decades, although recently there has been a trend in the opposite direction.

The major negative financial, administrative and emotional effects of HMOs, Medicaid, and, to a lesser extent, Medicare have been on primary care physicians, general internists, family medicine practitioners and pediatricians. With the advent of HMOs, the financial situation has not changed nearly as dramatically for specialists. Not that I think that the incomes of specialists have not changed at all, but there has been less of a change for them than for primary care physicians, internists and pediatricians. It is much easier for a cardiologist or oncologist or surgeon to survive a change of income going from $650,000 or more to $500,000, than for an internist or pediatrician to go from $250,000 to $150,000 while working as hard as possible.

Many physicians today feel that these changing conditions have resulted in insufficient time for them to do the best for their patients. They have to see more patients in a shorter time to generate sufficient income in their practices. Some doctors feel that their own financial pressures also influence the kinds of patients they see in their practices as providers. For example, it is not uncommon to read that some psychiatrists feel that they no longer "can afford" to offer talk therapy sessions (NYT). They only have time to make psychopharmacological assessments and fill out prescriptions for patients.

Many physicians, young and old, are either unwilling or unable to do the reams of paperwork and to make all of the phone calls necessary to give all the information required by HMOs, or to hire appropriate new staff to take on these tasks. Moreover, it is extremely time consuming to challenge decisions made by HMOs and other private insurers, and often only the physicians, not their staffs, can do so. Other physicians are just not willing to accept the low reimbursement rates from these HMOs or Medicare, and especially from Medicaid, a state-controlled program with consistently abysmal reimbursement rates to physicians.

These are the facts of modern medical practice and must be considered in planning for a decent reasonably priced medical care system in the United States that would be more generally available to us all. The pressures of time and money in modern medicine are enormous. Doctors cannot function successfully if they must see patients for only a limited time; listen to half or less of their stories, and feel they run the risk of coming to premature conclusions. All because they fear they run the risk of not making a reasonable income.

Really good doctors

For the doctors I know at Columbia-Presbyterian, mostly established older physicians, the strong and personal doctor–patient relationships have not changed substantially despite these new conditions. These dedicated physicians continue to spend as much time as necessary to optimally care for their patients. But their professional lives have become much more complex. For newer physicians, the landscape of private practice is continually changing and the future in terms of the practice conditions they must accept is unclear.

As I have said, there are, of course, still many really good doctors who have not fallen into any of the traps of the new medical care and reimbursement morass. They seem to have all the time in the world for their patients. I am fortunate enough to know some of the still excellent older physicians and excellent next-generation physicians, and to be cared for by several of them. I know that these doctors will always be focused on the best patient care; that they will always be truly attentive listeners, caregivers, and healers to all of their patients; that their egos will always be subservient to the needs of their patients; and that they will always be as smart, sensitive, and engaged with all of their patients as I know them to be. I consider them the true jewels of the profession.

Ed Leifer was one of those great doctors no matter whom he was caring for. He was completely focused on the problems of his patients. He listened to his patients, examined them, and then said what he had to say without much small talk or mincing words. Leifer believed in "tough love;" the patient had to act on his suggestions, take the medicines he prescribed, make the changes in life-style, long- or short-term, that he wanted. He was no soft, cuddly physician, and he lost patients because of his sometimes gruff demeanor, but to my mind he was a great physician. He exuded respect for the patient, and confidence in himself, and all of his patients trusted him with their health and their lives. But Ed Leifer, a general internist with an extraordinary reputation, would have done poorly financially in today's fee-for-service environment because he saw patients for too long a time and was constantly besieged by requests from them for even more of his time. He would not have appreciated or succumbed to the demands of HMOs, which affect time spent with patients in various ways, including time on the phone or computer, to expedite their "paperwork."

Physicians I know with traditional academic fee-for-service private practices at Columbia-Presbyterian have responded to the changes in medical insurance reimbursement by HMOs and Medicare and Medicaid in different ways. These physicians are not the usual internists or specialists in outside medical groups or working on their own. They all have appointments at Columbia University and most work within a faculty practice plan administered by the University. They also enjoy the benefits of tenured Columbia faculty, including generous University contributions to a retirement plan and tuition exemption benefits for their children. But they have been put under increasing financial pressure to generate adequate incomes by the changes in medical reimbursement patterns associated with the emergence of HMOs as well as decreases in Medicare and Medicaid reimbursement rates.

They have, at the same time, been subjected to taxes levied on their practice income by Columbia University and by their specific clinical departments and subspecialty divisions. Again, these taxes have been easier to bear for the doctors in the higher income groups than for internists and pediatricians making lower net incomes.

Because of these changing conditions, many older physicians at Columbia, as elsewhere, have retired early. Others have gone into medical administrative positions. The number of private practitioners doing general medicine and pediatrics has diminished at Columbia. Most physicians still in practice have modified their practices to accommodate the changes. The increased load of paperwork, phone calls, pre-approval planning for tests and hospital admissions demanded by many insurers today require additional secretarial and administrative help for which some physicians are not willing to pay. Because of these burdens, some practicing physicians and surgeons alike do not accept HMO patients except if they must as part of a faculty practice plan. Those who do accept HMO patients often have increased their staff by hiring additional secretarial help or administrators to help them deal with the increased paperwork for these patients, and either nurse practitioners or physician assistants to assist them with patient care.

Dr. Seth Feltheimer, a general internist in private practice at Columbia-Presbyterian, now has two secretaries and a physician assistant. He has made the choice to accept all patients who are insured, including those insured by HMOs and Medicare (but not Medicaid). He says he spends a significant amount of his time on the phone with insurers and staying current with the avalanche of changes in reimbursement policies from these sources. There are not many new generalists like Dr. Feltheimer in internal medicine at Columbia-Presbyterian.

Many practitioners, most of them specialists, either do not accept HMO patients, or accept only those HMO patients belonging to specific plans whom they are required to see as part of their participation in the Columbia faculty practice plan; some also do not accept Medicare for payment, except as they are required to do so as part of their participation in the faculty practice plan. They think Medicare reimbursement rates are too low. There are also many doctors who take no insurance at all. If you want to see these doctors, you have to pay out of pocket, or have good employer-provided or union-based or self-acquired private insurance that will reimburse you after you pay their fees.

Dubious activities

There has always been a small minority of doctors who have been involved in ethically dubious activities related to their patients. Because of the increased financial pressures of falling incomes from reduced patient care revenue, many more physicians have become involved in these activities than has been the case in the past. I personally know of no concrete instances of these kinds of activities, but rather rely on published news accounts, again largely in the NYT. I am referring to physicians who I believe are in obvious conflicts of interest between doing what is best for their patients on the one hand, and, on the other hand, complying with the demands of private arrangements with drug and device companies (and sometimes with hospitals) that may not be in the best interests of their patients.

Included in this category are physicians who are offered and accept a variety of financial incentives, such as large consultation fees and gifts and travel expenses, from drug and device companies to promote the use of new drugs, devices or procedures on their patients. One recent example reported in the media involved several prominent psychiatrists making hundreds of thousands of dollars from pharmaceutical companies for promoting the use of new psychoactive medications without demonstrated efficacy, while hiding their own financial interest.

Another recent example is the overuse of erythropoietin in oncology that cost patients and insurance plans millions of dollars, again involving collusion between drug companies and practitioners paid to give high doses of the drug to their patients. I do not think these are ethical ways of increasing physicians' incomes.

Most recently, the sale of drugs by physicians in their private offices at tremendous markups of prices has been reported (NYT). New for-profit companies have been created to buy drugs at lower prices from pharmaceutical companies and re-package these drugs to be sold in doctors' private offices, often at exorbitant price mark-ups, with the doctors and the companies sharing the profits. Abuses of drugs like oxycodone (Oxycontin) may be related to these new tactics and schemes that I consider highly unethical if not downright illegal. Drugs should not be re-packaged. They should be dispensed by pharmacies or in hospitals and, except in special medically justified cases, not in doctors' offices.

Other related problematic situations involve the use of a whole range of other new expensive anti-cancer medications which are only marginally effective but which are highly recommended by many oncologists at the urging of pharmaceutical companies, with remuneration to physicians for their use. Similarly, in other subspecialties, physicians collude with drug companies to favor the use of specific drugs for their own financial gain with no disclosure of conflicts of interest. The list goes on.

Scandals involving kickbacks to surgeons and hospitals for the use of defective devices in hip replacement surgery have been extensively reported in the press. The use of cardiac stents is another area of collusion; in this case, between physicians and the stent manufacturers, Several different brands of cardiac stents supplied by specific device companies have been reported to be associated with kickbacks to physicians and hospitals for their preferred use. Most recently, the vast overuse of stents without evidence of their benefit over routine medical therapy for certain cardiac conditions has been exposed (NYT). I think that physicians and hospitals involved in these activities should be severely reprimanded, but currently, they seem rarely affected by media disclosure.

There is recent Federal legislation that seeks to make all physician-drug company relationships disclosed and public. This is not enough. The only way these activities will be stopped is by passing laws that penalize physicians and the drug and device companies involved for these practices.

Physicians should also not be in a position to financially benefit from recommending specific tests or other services in which they have a personal financial interest. Financial gains to doctors from hospital or third party reimbursements for ordering tests and services or for arranging for more consultations provide an undesirable incentive for over-ordering tests and overdoing procedures and are a conflict of interest. This is another gray area in medicine. How much is a given doctor's referrals for testing and consultations being done for the patient's sake alone, how much of it has to do with defending the doctor from potential malpractice claims, and how much of it is related to increasing the overall money being reimbursed to the individual doctor or hospital? Because of these troubling ethical considerations, I believe that practicing physicians should not have ownership stakes in hospitals or in laboratories or in CAT scan or MRI machines or anything else that leads to financial incentives to maximize overuse for profit. Physicians should only be reimbursed for their own office-based or hospital-based direct services to the patient.

I am aware that there are currently many ethical and conflict-of-interest guidelines promulgated by the American Medical Association (AMA), states, hospitals and universities with respect to potential abuses by physicians, but they are largely ineffective and ignored. I am also well aware that there are many less restrictive conflict-of-interest guidelines and many dubious practices that pervade all other fields of endeavor, professional as well as commercial, in our society. So why should the medical profession be any different? My answer to that question goes back to my deep conviction that medicine is a calling, and that the practice of medicine must be held to the highest ethical standards, however high or low those standards are in other fields. What can be more bedrock fundamental than life itself and the entrusting of one person's life to another? I believe that only federal legislation will reduce unethical practices in medicine by making all the practices deemed unethical by professional guidelines illegal as well.

Most physicians earn much more than a living wage. Medical specialists and surgeons do particularly well financially. If physicians are not earning enough money, they can certainly find ethical ways to increase their incomes by changing the nature of their practices, expanding their practices, or charging higher fees for their services. They can also become more involved in administration or teaching for pay. Those physicians associated with medical schools and hospitals can often take on administrative or teaching responsibilities to supplement their incomes. Others can become hospitalists, salaried physicians who take care of hospitalized patients.

There are other legitimate ways in which practicing physicians can supplement their practice incomes. They can, of course, work longer hours. As specialists, they can work at multiple locations. They can also use their medical expertise to do consulting work for pharmaceutical or device companies if those activities do not raise conflict-of-interest issues regarding the care of their own individual patients. I think it is legitimate for physicians to participate in and be reimbursed for FDA-approved clinical trials under specified conditions in which they may receive a stipend from the study, even if the stipend comes from a pharmaceutical company, but they should not use their own patients in the trial because, again, the clinicians would have a conflict of interest: Are they using their patients because it is in the patients' best interest or for their own financial gain? This is often an ethically challenging situation especially when the drug companies sponsoring the trials are mainly interested in involving physicians who can contribute their own patients to these trials.

I have always done some extra work outside of my academic medicine position to supplement my income. Early in my academic career, I cared for hospital patients at night at other hospitals (so called "moonlighting"); later on, I earned money doing medical writing and editing. I have also consulted for drug and biotechnology companies in areas unrelated to my patient care activities, in accordance with the so-called "one day a week" policy at Columbia University which allows academics to engage in outside activities one day a week. I have also consulted for defense lawyers in some malpractice cases and for other lawyers in class action cases.

These and other kinds of activities involving being paid for medical expertise in arrangements free of conflict of interest issues are open to all physicians. I always knew that none of my activities could conflict with any aspect of my research and clinical responsibilities at Columbia. I also always disclosed all of my outside activities to the Columbia University administration annually.

Younger doctors

Becoming a physician and practicing medicine is a more difficult pursuit today than it has been in the past and, in addition to being personally gratifying, should be properly rewarded financially. All physicians deserve to be happy with their choices and their lives. But not at the expense of slip-shod medicine or ethically unacceptable financial arrangements with drug companies, device makers, hospitals or other doctors. The rationale given by many young doctors to justify the priority they put on high initial incomes is that they must pay off debts accrued during their education. This is a common situation today and the priority is understandable. As I have said before, I haven't seen many poor physicians. Future income will eventually pay off student loans. The desire to pay off debts quickly should not justify any compromise in the style of medicine that physicians practice that might lead to unethical activities like excessive testing, unnecessary hospitalizations, prescribing unnecessary medications and referring patients for consultations that are not in the best interests of their patients. I do think the government should find ways to reduce or, even better, forgive loans acquired by students who go into vital fields like medicine and teaching, but that is another issue.

It is also sad as well as a loss to society when bright young physicians choose more financially lucrative areas of practice over professional pursuits that might be more interesting and challenging to them, or areas of practice that address the more pressing needs of our society today, such as general medicine or pediatrics.

Today, more than ever, some young physicians may be influenced in their career choices by the fact that members of their generation in the financial industry and at big corporations and high tech companies are earning big money quickly and they want to do so as well. I think this is more difficult to accomplish in today's world of medicine. Feelings of envy and the relative financial success of people in other fields are no justification for young physicians to become focused on financial gain Their personal lives and professional gratification with their profession should suffice to sustain them until they achieve financial security in their chosen medical disciplines.

Generational changes in the lifestyles of doctors have also occurred recently. Younger physicians often do not wish to have their lives consumed by the intense mental and physical demands of medicine 24/7 that Dr. Leifer and others like him embraced in the past. There are still some such physicians but much fewer than there used to be. The inclination of many younger physicians to establish less intense medical practices that are in sync with a less pressured life style is understandable but sometimes involves a more limited commitment to patients on their part.

Fairly recent restrictive rules limiting the hours that house officers can work during their training and what they can do under current hospital regulations may have altered the perspective of these young physicians. These new rules are important and overdue positive reforms. However, one unintended consequence of these new regulations may be that they have made younger physicians less cognizant of the need for and the advantages of continuity of intensive patient care. They may, therefore, be more willing in this new environment to hand off and/or share care with other physicians and not take primary responsibility for the overall care of their patients to the extent that previous generations of physicians have.

Most older physicians I know, both general internists and medical specialists, have "coverage" of their patients by other physicians on some nights and weekends but continue to be the primary physicians for their patients long-term, guaranteeing continuity of care. But some physicians today work only 8–10 hour shifts and then routinely hand over the care of their patients to others. For example, there is a relatively new set of physicians, so-called hospitalists, doctors who only take care of hospitalized patients. They work shifts, and take care of the hospitalized patients of other physicians who do not want to take care of their ill hospitalized patients.

In my opinion, the emergence of hospitalists has compromised an important requirement for quality medical treatment: continuity of patient care. The patient is most often unknown to the hospitalist upon admission to the hospital, and is of no real concern to the hospitalist when he or she leaves the hospital. In this system, oversight of medications and follow-up are left to others. Certainly, hospitalists have little, if any, responsibility for what happens to the patients when the patients are discharged. This fragmentation of care increases the chances that patients will have to be re-admitted to the hospital with recurrent illness and results in increased costs of care as well as more poor outcomes. Hospitalists are here to stay, but the system they are part of needs to be reformed. Medical practice should not be fragmented into in-patient versus out-patient care; it should involve continuity of care with one primary physician at the helm at all times, as he or she integrates all aspects of the care of the patient.

Old school primary care physicians, including physicians in general medicine, general internists and pediatricians, and/or medical subspecialists who have a sizable subset of patients for whom they are the primary physician, are becoming a vanishing breed. Doctors are more and more often unavailable, especially at night and weekends. Many patients are now told to go to emergency rooms or to call 911 in emergencies.

How much responsibility for a patient's care should any one physician take? This is a difficult question to answer. Dr. Leifer, the best of physicians, may have set an impossibly high bar. It is also impossible for any physician to grade himself or herself as a physician personally. I certainly would find it hard to grade myself. How do doctors know how well they are doing or how much they should be doing for their patients? There is little assessment by peers, and patients are often too dependent on their doctors and/or not knowledgeable enough to be objective in even their lay evaluations. In any profession, it is difficult to monitor ones' own competence by oneself without some sort of outside review.

That is one reason why I never minded the peer review process as an integral part of my NIH research funding in my scientific career. At least it was an objective and detailed review of my activities, in this case, my research, by my peers. I had to pass muster; justify my activities; account for myself. Most physicians in practice never have to pass inspection and review. Unconcerned and even incompetent private practitioners can fly under any regulatory radar for most of their lives, unless their care involves truly egregious malpractice activity. Most academic physicians and teachers like I was, as well as doctors working in hospitals with academic affiliations, do get some limited feedback on their clinical activities from their departments, from their hospitals, and from fellow physicians, but not in a detailed way or with regularity.

Bad doctors

The overwhelming majority of doctors are at the very least competent, but there are some who are truly guilty of medical malpractice. When faced with two or more choices in the diagnosis or treatment of the patient, they will make the wrong choice, not out of malice, but out of ignorance and sloppy thinking. True malpractice occurs when the doctors' incompetence and/or lack of attention to detail in diagnosis and treatment do not meet the recognized standard of medical care and patients suffer physical and/or psychological adversity as a result. These doctors are appropriately sued for their poor medical care.

The legal system becomes dysfunctional in most medical malpractice cases because the huge financial stakes render it incompetent to deal with the truly important medical issues in each case. With these high financial stakes, lawyers, both on the side of patients and on the side of doctors and hospitals, try desperately to construct tricky "gotcha" arguments and reasoning in the courtroom to hammer home their respective points of view. The proper approach to malpractice cases should be to resolve them quickly and honestly, to assign appropriate blame when medically informed and objective parties decide that blame is due, and to see that the cases are not turned into multimillion-dollar circuses mostly benefiting lawyers. In the highly litigious, high financial stakes atmosphere that prevails today, many doctors are driven to practice defensive medicine and order unnecessary tests because of their fear of being sued.

I think most medical malpractice is unintentional and not truly criminal in nature and should be resolved by panels of medically knowledgeable objective "judges." Physicians should be more active participants, if not the final arbitrators and decision makers, in this process.

There are many other types of "bad doctors," in addition to those guilty of obvious malpractice. No one category describes them all. The worst ones to my mind are those who don't really care about their patients or how they treat them, and view them primarily as income-generating "clients." In this category are the private doctors in Medicare and Medicaid mills who often provide sub-standard medical care while making as much money as possible taking care of the elderly and the poor. These physicians, through overuse and fraud, game the Medicare/Medicaid system. They see as many patients as possible and provide only the most critical care necessary. They are often physicians at hospitals and private clinics in poorer neighborhoods (see NYT, Wykoff Hospital story recently).

Moving to the other end of the socioeconomic spectrum, there is also a small predatory subset of private practitioners who see primarily well-insured and/or very well-off patients and collect huge fees for their services. They include all types of physicians: internists, surgeons and all sub-specialists. They see patients too often; they do too many tests and procedures; they prescribe too many unnecessary, new and untested medications; and they vastly increase the cost of medical insurance and medical care for all. Most of these doctors get away with these activities because their patients, like most patients, do not know when these doctors are performing unnecessary, excessive and sometimes medically detrimental tests and services. Most of their patients think that these excesses of care and services are for their benefit and proof that they are getting superior care. They do not see the system as flawed and the high fees they are paying as unjustifiable.

Bad doctors are a small minority of physicians, but they are often able to practice their personally lucrative bad medicine for many years without detection. In the same way that I know that I am incompetent to judge for myself who would be a good lawyer or financial adviser for me, without expert advice, I understand that most non-physicians cannot easily judge who is a good physician and who is not.

The medical profession does an extraordinarily poor job of weeding out these predatory, sometimes incompetent physicians because of the generally poor monitoring of physicians. There is little or no continuous evaluation of physicians by medical boards, hospitals, states or the federal government. All you really have to do to continue to practice medicine is to pay the license fee in your state. Many bad doctors escape surveillance and practice unencumbered for years, even over their entire careers.

Best advice

We as patients have to try as hard as we can to identify the good doctors and stay away from the bad ones. My best advice is to focus on finding a single good doctor whom you trust to be your primary care physician. He or she should be either a primary care physician or an internist, either a general internist or a specialist who also has a substantial internal medicine practice and general medicine experience and interest. Rely on that one good doctor to send you to other good doctors he or she recommends. Try to find that one good doctor through a person who already has one, although that is not always a foolproof approach and some trial and error corrections may be necessary. If you are referred to specialists for every little thing and feel that your primary care doctor is primary in name only because he or she does not seem to be at the helm of your case in coordinating the input of others, you may want to seek out another primary care physician who will give you a more secure sense of being in good hands.

When you come into a doctor's office and the doctor is either on the phone; or talking to his nurse or secretary; or telling you or them about his or her latest cultural, political, financial or social experience; or blabbing away about anything that isn't related to your care, you should get out of that doctor's care as soon as you can. When you come into a doctor's office, you should be the sole focus of the doctor's attention and your concerns and care should be the only things of importance to that doctor while you are there. That is the covenant of the doctor-patient relationship.

CHAPTER SIXTEEN

The Business of Medicine

The medical care system in the United States is currently in crisis. The major reason for this crisis is that medicine has become much more of a business than a profession. As my friend Dr. Jordan Cohen puts it, "There has been a loss of professionalism and an increase in commercialism in medicine today." Dr. Arnold Relman, an excellent physician whom I have previously mentioned, and who was for many years the editor-in-chief of the New England Journal of Medicine, has been an early and continuing critic of the increased influence of businessmen and private investors in medical care. His and many others' warnings about the negative effects of an unbridled medical care for-profit industry on medical care today may have been heard but have largely gone unheeded and ignored.

As I have said before, not much has changed in the basic compact between good doctors and their individual patients. However, although doctors are still the same healers and empathetic caretakers as in the past, the intrusion of commercialism in obtaining medical care has radically complicated the relationships between doctors and patients.

The first question we are asked today when we seek a new physician's care by telephone is not "How can I help you?", which we might expect, but, "What kind of insurance do you have?" Or, on reaching the doctor's office, we may be informed that the doctor doesn't accept any insurance, period. If the doctor doesn't accept our insurance, or any insurance, we have to grapple with whether we want to incur the often sizable additional costs to pay the doctor out of pocket in the hope that we will be reimbursed for some portion of our cash outlay from the insurance we do have.

Another characteristic of the new milieu of medical care is that because of the increased perceived value of every minute of a doctor's time, it is considerably more difficult today than it used to be to contact a new doctor, or indeed our own longstanding doctors, even in an emergency. There are new constraints on when you can reach your doctor by phone or by appointment. Although they are hugely important to health care delivery, nurse practitioners, physician-assistants, as well as office managers often make it more difficult for the average patient to access the doctor directly. Unless you're seriously ill, it's almost always, "The doctor will get back to you," which more times than not means either not the same day or that you will have to call again.

Today, in addition to those of us with health insurance, there are over 40 million people in the United States with no coverage at all. The uninsured depend on care in crowded emergency rooms and public clinics that fall far short of delivering either timely medical treatment or continuity of care. Patients die in the United States every day because they are denied medical care due to lack of insurance. The book, "The Healing of America," by T. R. Reid details the reasons for this unconscionable problem in the United States. Simply put, we are the only democracy in the developed world without available universal health care. This is because we Americans and our elected political representatives have been unwilling to buy into a medical care and insurance system that provides all of us with care while controlling costs in any of the various ways that other countries like England, Canada, France, Germany, Taiwan and many others have successfully done. Unlike these other countries, we are unwilling to have a system that pays for all physician services, all hospital care and most medications for all, and, most importantly, allays our anxieties about being denied medical care when we need it because we can't afford it.

In other countries with universal health care the costs of medical care are controlled by government policy. In the United States, doctors and hospitals and drug and device makers largely charge what they want to. Then health insurance companies including HMOs transfer these costs of coverage to us, their customers, routinely adding additional charges to their premiums to ensure profits for themselves and their investors.

Many hospitals exploit the disorganized American health care system by inflating their charges to maximize reimbursement in various manipulative and/or dishonest ways; for example, they often add unnecessary and undocumented extra charges to their bills. And ideally there should be no big strictly for-profit hospital corporations with investors at all because they only increase overall medical costs, but these entities continue to expand and proliferate. It turns the hospitals into businesses, not primarily places for care.

Pharmaceutical companies also exploit the disorganized American health care system with the result that the costs of drugs to everyone, even those of us on Medicare and Medicaid, are hugely inflated and the companies' profits continue to grow, largely unregulated. The abuses of drug companies in the US are legion both in their marketing strategies as well as in their pricing. These companies are an especially onerous drag on the American health care consumer, always marketing new and often unnecessary products every day. They have huge marketing budgets. They have representatives flooding doctors' offices daily.

They also have misleading and unregulated ads on almost every network television news show as well as other network and cable shows. It is difficult for the busy physician, let alone patients, to distill the truth about new advertised drugs. "Ask your doctor if you need X (a new medicine)," is the common mantra of these commercials. This advertising is very glib, often misleading or false and scientifically undocumented. It should be forbidden. The whole idea that patients should be asking or telling their doctors what to prescribe is ludicrous. That is the doctor's job. If you don't think your doctor is capable of doing this job, find a new doctor. And beware of doctors who are quick to acquiesce to your requests. These doctors do not empower patients; they shirk their responsibilities as doctors to direct their patients' medical treatment. All of the marketing activity of the pharmaceutical industry costs enormous amounts of money, and the costs are passed on directly to all of us as health care consumers.

Drug companies are charging too much for their medications. Using various strategies, they are also constantly fighting to keep cheaper generic versions of their brand name drugs (same drugs without the brand name) off the market after the patents for their more expensive brand name versions expire; this often occurs because generic drug companies have negotiated with, or have been paid off by, the larger patent-owning pharmaceutical company to have the generic drug version disappear or become less available to drug plans. This practice should be illegal. In just this past year, three of my own medications, which were available through my insurance plan as generic versions ($10 per month), were discontinued by manufacturers and only became available as their brand name versions ($25 a month). Companies producing brand name drugs have also taken little if any responsibility for assuring that the adequate flow of vital drugs continues after their patents expire or after they become less profitable; this situation accounts for the recent well-documented shortages of several vital anti-cancer drugs and other medicines (NYT).

Our government, which pays for Medicare and Medicaid coverage with our tax money, is prevented by law from negotiating lower prices with drug companies to lower the costs of medications for Medicare or Medicaid patients, and the Medicare Part D program available to Medicare recipients does nothing to change this. The program often pays the costs of brand name drugs if no generic equivalents are available (in many cases because the generic drug companies have been paid to have them disappear), or because physicians, despite the existence of generic alternatives on the market, prescribe the drugs under their brand names. This is outrageous. In addition, there are there so many different Medicare Part D drug coverage plans to choose from that it is almost impossible for any patient to figure out the best one for him or her. The Medicare Part D program has been a boondoggle for drug companies and an enormously crushing expense to the federal government and consumers.

Device makers constitute another group of largely unregulated for-profit companies that have contributed heavily to the rising price of health care because of the constantly rising prices of both their older products as well as their novel often untested and unregulated newer ones. Some of these new scanning and diagnostic and surgical machines are indeed better for patient care, but device company representatives are also hawking newer and slicker versions of older machines as well as other new devices that are often wasteful and unnecessary and that have not been shown to improve outcomes.

I met a 25-year old guy on a plane a couple of years ago who was flying around the world selling new hardware for use in spinal cord operations. He worked for a small company. He had no medical training or background. He was a salesman. It was not that the old hardware he was seeking to replace was outmoded. It was just that his company had changed things a bit to allegedly improve the way spinal cord surgery was done and how spines are surgically repaired. He was paid only on commission for every sale he made, each of which was in the tens of thousands of dollars. The money was great for him. Was he trained to evaluate the hardware? No. Did he care whether it was needed? No. Did his new device work better than existing devices? He didn't know. He was only trained to demonstrate the new device, even to surgeons in surgical operating rooms, and to sell them. It was just another great business in the business of medicine. He was completely unregulated in his activities, as are most device makers and their representatives.

For decades, the Federal Drug Administration, the FDA, despite its mandate as a regulator of safety and efficacy, sadly, has been an inadequate overseer of the many problems caused by drug and device makers. Many drugs, and devices, including certain hip replacement devices, cardiac pacemakers and defibrillators, have not been identified early enough as defective and dangerous. Political interference in the activities of the FDA, the lack of adequate personnel and inadequate federal funding have been the major reasons for this. Drug and device makers that the FDA is mandated to regulate have provided much of the agency's limited funding. This is an unacceptable conflict of interest. Dr. Margaret Hamburg is a superb new leader of the agency but she needs expanded government financial support to restore its reputation. Federal funding must be increased to increase the manpower, facilities and independence of the agency, and political interference must be stopped if the FDA is to restore its mandated regulatory authority and the efficiency it needs to protect the public from the increasing number of potentially dangerous and unnecessary drugs and devices.

The costs of Medicare and Medicaid, the largest insurance providers in the US, continue to rise annually due to the largely inadequate oversight by federal regulators and politicians of reimbursement in these programs to doctors, hospitals, drug companies, and device makers. Several estimates, including those of Dr. Saul Berwick, recently the temporary administrator of the Centers for Medicare and Medicaid Services (CMS), indicate that 20–30% of the costs in Medicare are due to overpayments, waste and fraud. A recent Institute of Medicine report indicates that an estimated $750 billion a year is wasted on unnecessary and inefficient activities in the American health care system, representing 20–30% of our total health care costs.

There are clearly inequities in Medicare and private insurance reimbursement. Many physicians performing procedures, especially surgeons and other specialists, are being reimbursed too well by Medicare and private insurance carriers. Similarly, drug and device makers are paid too much. On the other hand, reimbursement to general practitioners, general internists and pediatricians is often inadequate; they are paid much less for their time and services. Too many unnecessary tests and procedures are being done.

The politicization of Medicare reimbursement policies has been astounding. Instead of being run by doctors and competent independent regulators, Medicare is run primarily by appointees approved by politicians; and many of these politicians are lobbied by, and, in turn, support the interests of specific health care groups who contribute heavily to their campaigns. These special interest groups include drug and device makers, the AMA, and the American Hospital Association (AHA). People like Dr. Berwick, who favor reform and are immensely qualified to run the system, are marginalized and rejected. Berwick recently resigned when it became clear he had no chance of being appointed by Congress as the permanent director of CMS. He was criticized and became unacceptable to politicians because he had praised the idea of universal health care and the government-run British health care system.

The fee-for-service for-profit practice of medicine has always existed in the United States. But never has it been so ruthlessly exploited as today. The business of medicine has overtaken the profession. Overall, health care is about 18% of our total economy, much greater than that of other countries, but we have less successful medical outcomes. The medical sector has taken its lessons from the financial sector in our country with disastrous consequences for patients. Private investors and venture capitalists have turned health insurance companies into financial behemoths. Most medical groups, hospitals, pharmaceutical companies and device makers are driven by the profit motive with little thought about the best and most affordable medical care for patients. The primary goal of the system is not to deliver better or more efficient care to patients, but to make money, as much money as possible for the private business sector. The pressure for big profit margins for investors is the main driving force and has driven up the cost of medical insurance for most of us by leaps and bounds over the last few decades.

Every patient is understandingly most concerned with his or her own care, and relatively less interested in finding solutions to the larger problems of cost and fragmentation of care in the system as a whole. The rich, many trade union members, workers with adequate employer-generated health care, and government workers with guaranteed and satisfactory medical plans, primarily favor the status quo for medical insurance in America. These groups present a formidable obstacle to any progress in achieving a system of more widespread care for all, even though most of their benefits are unsustainable over time without a greater contribution from them in the future.

Likewise, senior citizens, also receiving adequate care at reasonable prices through Medicare, do not generally favor changes in the system that they feel might result in decreased benefits or increased costs to them in the future, when in fact an unchanged Medicare system is also unsustainable over time. Meanwhile, most patients not eligible for union or employer plans, and not eligible for Medicare or Medicaid, are paying too much for medical care; or cannot find affordable care; or have no medical care other than that which is available in emergency rooms or free clinics. That there are over 40 million uninsured citizens in the United States is a horrific statistic. This is a national tragedy, and it has become one of the greatest ethical, social and financial challenges that America has ever faced.

My medical insurance

Medical insurance for my family and myself has always been a major concern for me, as it is for almost everybody. Columbia University benefits are extremely generous and, to the best of my knowledge, are unsurpassed by other educational institutions. While I was an active faculty member at Columbia University, the insurance plan was reasonably priced. The costs of care were shared between Columbia and me. After I retired, however, I became quite uncomfortable with my insurance coverage because of changes in federally-based insurance coverage and reimbursement policies.

I was primarily covered by Medicare, but Medicare does not pay for many services; it only pays for 80% of most services and it does not pay for drugs unless one acquires Medicare Part D coverage. I could never completely comprehend the value to me of Medicare Part D coverage, since no one Part D plan covered all of my medicines, and since it has huge financial holes in it that require significant financial outlays. For these reasons, I enrolled in a Columbia University Retiree Medical Plan which had several options, including different supplemental insurance carriers that covered costs not met by Medicare, and drug coverage. I opted for the most complete plan available. It is expensive, but it does provide full drug coverage, a costly item, with reasonable drug co-pays: $10 for generics, $25 for brand name drugs. Not bad.

In early November 2007, at age 72, I was becoming a bit panicky about renewing my medical insurance since information was hard to come by at the time and the available retiree medical plans were rapidly changing. I failed to get my original contact person at the Columbia Benefits Office when I called in early November. Instead, I talked with another young woman and I told her that I was worried about my health insurance coverage since I still had not heard from the benefits office about my retirement medical options for January 1, 2008 and it was already November 2007. She told me what I had been hearing for the last six months: "We are finalizing a plan."

She also told me that I was lucky that they were coming up with a retiree health plan because "a lot of large corporations are not offering any health plans for retirees anymore or dropping them." I hung up. I called again very shortly thereafter and talked with my original contact person. She was calm and competent-sounding and I told her of my earlier conversation with her associate and she apologized, but said there still was no plan. The new plan was "still being finalized." She suggested I call CBA/EBPA, the company in charge of administering and billing for the plan, to find out the details.

The first lady I talked to at CBA/EBPA transferred me to the lady in charge of medical benefits for retirees who told me that they had no final information about the Retiree Health Plan options for the next year. So next, I talked again to the Benefits Office, the third time that month. This time, I asked to speak to a higher up in the office who was knowledgeable about the Retiree Health Plan. He told me "we are finalizing a plan." I told him I was concerned. He calmly said, "Not to worry. We will have a plan going out, not next week, the week after." I thanked him for his time and hung up. Eventually, I received the details of the 2008 plan and my wife and I were enrolled. I'm sure the people I talked to in the above account thought I was overreacting. And, in retrospect I see that I was.

In truth, everyone I spoke to was steadfast and confident in the knowledge that there was no problem in finalizing a plan that would go into effect in 2008. What was happening to me was that I was being revisited by my worst health care nightmare that had been set off originally by an alarming experience that I had with my primary insurance carrier not long after a diagnosis of my colon cancer many years before.

I have been particularly anxious about my health coverage since 1988, when one Friday, late in the day, I received a letter from Oxford Health Plans, the primary insurer through my Columbia insurance then, that said my coverage had lapsed and was no longer in effect, and that I was no longer covered by their company. At that time, on that day, the news was a catastrophe for me. I was being treated for colon cancer then with intravenous medication during expensive weekly hospital visits. I was also in danger of having a relapse of my cancer that may have involved additional treatments such as operations and other medicines. In this short letter received on that Friday afternoon, I was being told that my insurance was cancelled. I was stunned. I had a very unpleasant and anxious weekend.

On the following Monday, I called Oxford. The lady I talked to there calmly told me, after reviewing my records, that my insurance coverage was indeed intact with Oxford. No problem. "It was a computer glitch," she explained. Nothing more. I was not happy. I asked how that could happen. She said: "It just happens." I asked, "Don't you check it out before you send letters to people cancelling their insurance?" She said, "No, the letter is generated automatically by the computer. We believe the computer."

I had been sobered and disillusioned by this experience. What do other employees and retirees do when they have medical insurance problems, if I, as a long-term physician involved in the medical care system, despite my best efforts, could never rest assured that my insurance would not be be disrupted or cancelled?

The big picture

My medical insurance story pales in comparison to those of so many others in America who cannot afford health care for their families and themselves. More and more in our present economy, as insurance is becoming more expensive, employers, the major source of health care financing for many Americans, are either curtailing their contributions drastically or no longer providing any coverage at all. The latest wrinkle is offering medical insurance with extremely high deductibles at lower monthly costs, another dangerous untested approach.

Many thousands of Americans are dying needlessly today because they cannot obtain adequate medical care. Examples abound of uninsured patients who have died with chronic diseases like lupus or hypertension or diabetes because they lacked adequate continuous care. They are people who would have survived if they had received proper care, or if they had lived in countries with universal health care.

A recent study of poorer patients, some of whom were randomly assigned to receive Medicaid coverage while others were not, demonstrated that by the end of the study those with access to Medicaid were healthier than those without access; presumably this result was obtained because patients who had Medicaid coverage sought care more often and received successful treatment for their health care problems (NYT 2011). It seems obvious: those of us without access to care because we can't afford it will be sicker and in greater danger of dying, and less able to live normal productive lives. Health insurance is critical to receiving adequate health care. We must find a way to provide affordable health insurance for everyone in the United States.

The lack of affordable health care in the United States for so many of our citizens is hard to accept, but what makes it even more difficult for me to accept is my belief that at its best American health care is the best health care in the world. We have the best doctors, the best hospitals, and the best drug and device industries. Major medical breakthroughs continue to come primarily from American medical research, both basic research and clinical studies. For example, cholesterol-lowering agents were developed by American scientists and physicians.

American medical practice also rapidly incorporates the most important recent advances in diagnosis and treatment based on discoveries made around the world. I have been particularly impressed with strides made in laparoscopic surgery, initially developed in Europe and now widely practiced here, which have resulted in shorter hospital stays and less morbidity for patients.

Sophisticated diagnostic testing and excellent updated medical and surgical treatments are available all over the United States. Yet the promise of all of these improvements in health care remains limited as long as there are so many of our citizens who are uninsured and whose lives will not be saved or made more manageable because adequate care is not available to them. This situation is just unfair and even more frustrating when one thinks about the fact that so many research advances in the development of newer methods in diagnosis and treatment have been *publically* funded in our country. Now, instead of benefitting the public at large, these advances have become part and parcel of the commercialization of medicine in the United States.

CHAPTER SEVENTEEN

Solutions

The goal of medicine in the United States should be excellent and affordable health care for everyone by dedicated caring physicians. We are the richest nation on earth and can achieve this goal with an appropriate political climate and a revised equitable system of taxation and regulation. One class care, such as Medicare for all, should be our goal, at the very least.

To achieve this goal it is imperative that our health care system control the costs of medical care. Strong government regulation of health care costs is the only way this has been accomplished in all of the countries with universal health care to date: countries like England, Germany, Canada, France, Taiwan and Japan, and others (T.R. Reid book). This is not to say that any of these countries have been able to find easy solutions to the rising costs of medical care. They continue to struggle as we do with the escalating costs of care as larger aging populations with more health problems and as more sophisticated and expensive technologies appear. In all of these countries, the governments have ongoing battles with health care providers, especially doctors, who in most instances have seen their incomes reduced substantially with the advent of universal care.

Government programs in these countries have also been forced to revise the availability of some kinds of care deemed less essential or inadvisable, and to exclude payment for expensive testing and therapies that are not proven to be beneficial. They also have a problem of long waiting times, usually for non-emergency services. But in the end, they all have universal health care and its overwhelming societal advantages. Every patient has a doctor; every patient is cared for; every citizen is secure in knowing his or her medical care will be there when he or she needs it. And contrary to the myth circulated in American public opinion, while some patients may wait for certain elective medical and surgical services, emergency care is readily available in these countries. No one dies because medical care is denied due to a lack of insurance, as occurs every day in our country. And the international ratings for care in these countries by most measures are far superior to ratings for care in the United States.

There is no way there will be a solution to the health care crisis in the United States without significantly increased government regulation. In almost all countries with universal health care, the government stringently controls reimbursement to doctors and hospitals as well as the cost of drugs, devices and diagnostic tests. In every country with universal health care, the cost of care for individual services is not left up to private interests, health providers, or private insurers. Despite the desirability of universal health care, given the current political and social climate in the United States, I do not believe that it is possible in the very near future to establish the conditions necessary to achieve truly universal health care here.

The Affordable Care Act

We as a society elected Barack Obama in 2008 with the hope that he would rescue us from impending financial ruin and end our useless wars. He immediately addressed these issues but, at the same time and at considerable political risk, he also focused on achieving health care reform. He and the Democratic Congress embraced the message that everyone deserves affordable health care, and that it is a moral as well as a social and financial imperative to do so. Miraculously, Nancy Pelosi and the Democratic Congress passed the Affordable Care Act (ACA) in 2009. In passing this landmark bill, the best bill it could pass with total Republican opposition, the Obama administration tried to begin to solve the problem of insuring more than 40 million Americans without health insurance, and to curtail the high costs and abuses of the current system. Despite its modest goals, the implementation of the new ACA continues to be fought tooth and nail at every possible level by conservatives and various special interest groups.

The bill requires that health care insurers enroll all who apply for insurance coverage, regardless of their history of prior illnesses; prohibits insurers from dropping people from coverage once insured; and prohibits insurers from setting any lifetime limitation to their health care insurance benefits. These provisions at the heart of the bill end major abuses of insurance providers. There is also a provision for medical coverage of dependents under age 26 in the bill that brings tremendous relief on many levels to millions of American families. These are all provisions that are currently in effect, but go largely unappreciated by many in the public at large. President Obama and the Democrats get little credit for them. I don't know why.

The Affordable Care Act has two major goals. The first is to provide medical care to most of our currently uninsured 40 million plus citizens; and second, to do so at affordable rates that will, over the long-term, rein in our individual and governmental health care spending. As I have said before, the health care sector spending in the US represents about 18% of our national economy. Our expenditures for health care are much greater than those of other developed countries, most of which spend less than half as much per person as we do.

A single payer system, an expansion of Medicare in some form, would have been the most efficient way of providing cheaper and more efficient coverage for every citizen, the most important goal. But this single payer government program was unacceptable to the vast private for-profit health insurance industry because it would have meant its imminent demise. It was never a viable political option.

The next best way to try to lower costs and provide wider care would have been through a "public option," an option to obtain insurance provided by the federal government for any one who either did not have and/or cannot get private insurance, and is not now eligible for Medicare or Medicaid. This government-sponsored public option would compete with private insurance companies on an even footing for all new available customers, and this competition would optimally lower individual health care costs. But the realistic prospect that the lower costs required to administer the public option would enable it to out-compete private health insurers and possibly lead to their eventual demise triggered vehement opposition to the public option. Insurance companies lobbied Congress and the White House and managed to defeat the plan. The defeat of the public option was a major disappointment to many of us who thought the public option was the only politically acceptable and effective way at this time in this country to insure more people, lower costs, and help curb the profits and influence of private health care insurers.

Instead, what was finally included in the bill were weaker "exchanges," options to buy insurance provided by individual states for people who could not otherwise obtain private health insurance. This is a less acceptable and less effective way of reducing the costs of care because the state legislatures will have the right to configure these policies and modify the insurance coverage in their own ways; some states have already made it clear that they intend to obstruct the exchange process because it will cost them money to establish these exchanges and/or because they don't like the idea of government getting in the way of the business of private insurance. According to the ACA, eventually, if the states do not set up appropriate exchanges, federal government exchanges to serve this function would be established. This all seems like a long drawn-out process, and, indeed, the changes are scheduled to kick in over several years, beginning in 2014. The exchanges as currently conceived will probably insure fewer people than the initially proposed federal public option would have, will probably cover mainly poorer and sicker citizens not currently eligible for Medicare or Medicaid, and may not compete well with private insurers in any meaningful way.

The most controversial part of the Affordable Care Act is the requirement that every citizen is insured. People who cannot afford insurance on their own will be insured by expanded Medicaid coverage. But the ACA mandates that health insurance be obtained by everyone else who is not covered but who can afford to pay health insurance,. Those who can afford health insurance but do not obtain it must pay a financial penalty, a tax. There is no loophole. The mandate would theoretically insure that almost all, if not all, people in the US would have insurance coverage and that we as a nation would finally have a health care system in which our population would be close to universally insured.

This mandate is absolutely necessary for the ACA to work for several reasons. Most importantly, it makes the ACA more palatable to private health care insurers by providing them with many millions of new customers, mainly relatively healthier younger people. These relatively healthier younger people reduce the average cost of care per person paid by the insurers. The insurers need these relatively healthier younger people paying premiums into their programs in order to lower their net costs per patient and to better compete with new government-sponsored plans. Only if enough relatively healthy and young new payers buy insurance and increase their revenues without proportionately increasing their costs can the insurers reduce their costs per patient.

Secondly, without this mandate that everyone who can afford insurance obtain it, uninsured patients will continue to overuse emergency rooms, hospital wards and public clinics as their primary source of care. Because these overcrowded and expensive facilities are publicly funded, they constitute an increased tax burden for the rest of us; we are paying the medical bills for many people who should be paying for themselves and are not doing so. Additionally, emergency care is transient and variable and is not nearly as effective as care by primary care physicians and medical groups in which the histories of patients are known to their doctors and in which preventive services are provided. Preventive care and continuity of care, respectively, are necessary to avoid and treat illnesses like chronic obesity, diabetes, and heart disease; they are likewise necessary to forestall progression of, and prevent death from, a host of other diseases that could be detected early and treated.

Conservatives and their allies have taken the legal position that it is unconstitutional for any American to be forced to pay for health care insurance, and, therefore, cannot be mandated to do so under the so-called Commerce Clause of the Constitution. The issue of the mandate had been debated in the lower courts and in the preliminary discussion of the law at the Supreme Court, the conservative justices on the Court showed little concern regarding the importance of mandated health insurance coverage as it relates to the national health care crisis in our country. Justice Scalia asked: "What about broccoli?" He compared penalizing people who did not buy health insurance that they could afford with penalizing people for not buying broccoli. He was suggesting that forcing people to obtain health insurance would establish a precedent that would go so far as to allow the government to penalize us for not buying anything else they wanted us to buy, including broccoli. This is a slippery-slope theory with which many legal scholars disagree. From their perspective, health insurance is a uniquely national and urgent issue extensively involving interstate commerce and can be mandated under the Commerce Clause.

Imagine, this is an argument about penalizing people who don't want to pay for health care insurance that they can afford, even though they know that their health care is paid for by the rest of us when they get sick. What has happened to our sense of individual responsibility and to our sense of fair play that requires us to act for the good of the society as a whole?

Surprisingly, despite the conservative majority on the Supreme Court, the mandate, together with most of the rest of the Affordable Care Act, was upheld by the Court on June 28, 2012. Chief Justice John Roberts saved the mandate and the Act by voting with the four more liberal justices. He justified the mandate on the basis that Congress had the power to tax and viewed the mandate as a tax. (However, at the same time, Roberts did vote with the conservatives that the mandate violated the Commerce Clause.) If Roberts had not joined the liberal wing to approve the mandate, the entire Affordable Care Act would have been overturned. If the mandate had been overturned, it would have been the final nail in the coffin for the Act since if there were no mandate, there would be no penalty for those who chose not to obtain insurance. With less money coming into the system, insurance companies would have had no incentive to support the other provisions of the law.

The Affordable Care Act, also called the Obama bill or Obamacare, is not nearly close to all that we really need to do to comprehensively address the medical care and insurance crisis in America, but it makes a good start. We are all at risk for illness and need coverage. The idea that nearly universal health coverage is being mandated and there will be financial penalties for people who do not have such coverage but can afford it is only reasonable.

Despite its passage and the Supreme Court decision that it is constitutional, the ACA is still being fought by the right wing as "socialism." Some of the resistance to health care reform on the part of some of our citizens comes from ignorance of the role the government already plays in health care and insurance, as was illustrated by a sign at a Tea Party rally demanding that the government keep its hands off the sign-bearer's Medicare. The House of Representatives with a Republican majority voted in July 2012 to repeal the ACA, but the repeal effort died in the Senate.

Over the three years since its passage, the ACA has failed to win over the enthusiastic, or even lukewarm, support of many people who are part of different constituencies. The administration must do a much better job of convincing the American people of its benefits. Those lacking enthusiasm for the bill include many in the health care industry who want the status quo, those who already have insurance that meets their own needs and is paid for through employer health plans or union health plans or the government (Medicare/Medicaid), as well as those who already have, because they can afford to have, insurance on their own. Joining the ranks of people who have little enthusiasm for the ACA are many of those who, as I have already pointed out, do not have health insurance because they don't want to pay for it, not because they can't afford it. So the reasons for resistance to health care reform vary. Medicare recipients are afraid their benefits will decrease as more people are being supported by government plans. And many Americans who think they already have good medical insurance and many who can afford it on their own aren't willing to give that same medical security to others who don't have good health insurance and can't afford it on their own.

A sizable number of senior citizens who already have government coverage through Medicare don't want to see their own safety net for health care extended in any form to their own children and grandchildren lest their own care be affected in any way. They are too selfish and/or uninformed to see that extending government health insurance to all through a public option would have actually benefited them because it would have been the most efficient way to control medical costs, including their own, in the health care system as a whole. Government health care programs such as Medicare, Medicaid and programs under the Veterans Administration have much lower administrative costs than private insurance carriers, and do not have to generate profits for investors the way insurance companies and for-profit hospitals do. The Affordable Care Act does mandate that at least 80% of revenues generated by insurance companies must now be spent on patient care and not on administrative services or profits to investors, a welcome change from past practices.

The Affordable Care Act also has some other excellent provisions which would lower costs by lowering reimbursement rates to certain physicians and hospitals for services they are currently financially incentivized to do, such as CAT scans and MRIs, the overuse of which carries increased medical risks and costs to patients, as well as for other laboratory tests and procedures. For example, as mentioned earlier, it has recently been shown that most cardiac stents are unnecessary, but with doctors and hospitals getting thousands of dollars for each procedure, only lower reimbursement rates will curtail unnecessary treatments of this kind.

Another excellent provision of the ACA calls for the establishment of a panel of medical experts to determine the validity of Medicare and Medicaid costs and to suggest changes to get the prices of services under control, rather than to continue the present system of having costs regulated primarily by bureaucrats and politicians beholden to special interest groups like drug and device makers, hospitals, and the AMA. If this provision is maintained as the bill goes through modifications, it would be a critical new control point for these programs and assure that professionals rather than politicians determine what changes in reimbursement policies need to be made. Currently, fraud and abuse in Medicare and Medicaid programs costs taxpayers billions of dollars annually.

Hopefully, the day will come when the pharmaceutical industry is more tightly regulated, especially regarding the cost of drugs. The chicanery surrounding the passage of Medicare Part D during the Bush administration, a gift to the drug industry paid for by plunging the nation into further untenable debt, is too mind-boggling to be summarized here. Suffice it to say that the industry has had its way politically, limiting the ability of the government even with our huge government programs like Medicare and Medicaid to negotiate drug prices with the companies. This must change. Drug costs are too high.

Similarly, the costs of services and the profit margins for tests, such as blood tests and genetic tests, should be regulated more tightly, not only with respect to reimbursement by Medicare and Medicaid, but more broadly for those tests done outside of these government programs.

Preventive services should be covered in all health plans, both public and private. Appropriate prenatal care, women's care, vaccinations, diet and health care advice should be built into all plans. Some preventive services are currently required by the ACA to be covered by private insurers.

Dental care is deteriorating for many children and adults in the United States, primarily because of its expense. It should be provided more broadly by insurance plans, and its costs more tightly controlled.

Preventive as well as emergent dental care, currently too expensive for the average citizen, should be available to everyone at reasonable costs.

A good health care delivery system would ideally involve the designation of a single person, a combination of case manager and ombudsman, for each of us; either a medical administrator or a social worker or a physician or a nurse practitioner or physician assistant to coordinate all aspects of our individual care, to avoid the fragmentation of care so common in medical practice today. Programs already exist where this practice already occurs, but it should be more generally applied. In addition, public health initiatives such as programs to fight our most common medical problems today, especially in the young, such as obesity and diabetes, should also be dramatically expanded.

And finally, eventually, hospital costs and physician reimbursement, especially for medical and surgical specialists, ophthalmologists, dermatologists, radiologists, and anesthesiologists currently operating both within and outside of Medicare and Medicaid, will need to be regulated by the states or the Federal government to reduce overall costs. In addition, I would hope that all physicians, especially primary care physicians, internists and pediatricians, would eventually be enticed, by appropriate reimbursements, to participate in Medicare and Medicaid. In my heart, I think that eventually there must be price controls placed on all physician services and hospital costs for the greater good of our economy and our society. However, the chances of any, much less all, of the above listed proposals happening in the near future in our current political environment is close to zero because politicians backed by special interest groups will fight any government-mandated cost controls. Senate Republicans in particular have vowed not to confirm anyone with cost-cutting and progressive views like those of the excellent Dr. Saul Berwick as permanent head of the Medicare/Medicaid programs.

The battles with private insurers, private doctors, private hospitals, pharmaceutical companies and device makers to contain and regulate health care costs in the private sector will continue into the future, and I am doubtful that such truly comprehensive regulation will occur in my lifetime. Not with our current political climate. Our society is not yet ready to meet our social and ethical obligations to provide adequate health care to all of our citizens at reasonable costs.

But I am hopeful that the future of medicine will include a shift from its present convoluted fee-for-service system with individual payments in individual private practices to more integrated multidisciplinary health care delivery systems in which physicians, nurse practitioners, physician assistants and their support staffs, and health care providers in many different medical and surgical fields, are grouped together and their activities integrated. These so-called "bundled care" systems have been shown to be more effective in delivering good medical care while reducing the overall cost of medical care. These "accountable care organizations" exist throughout the United States but they must become the dominant model for health care delivery and be publicly supported. More importantly, these new models must be accepted and supported by the medical establishment as well as the public as we try different paths in searching for the best medicine.

CHAPTER EIGHTEEN

Changing Times

There has been a sea change in priorities in the United States over the last 30 years. The top one percent of the population now dominates our economy. Money talks; morality matters little. We have become more and more entangled in the stranglehold of unfettered capitalism. The political reach of the rich and powerful in industry has never been greater. The financial industry now constitutes about 20% of our economy. The health care industry approaches another 18%, a much greater share than in any other country. The defense industry with its multi-billion dollar defense contractors; multinational corporations primarily based in the United States; and the oil and gas industry have all expanded their scope. From the operation of prisons to the waging of war, privatization is the order of the day. Privatization is threatening the critical lifeblood of public education.

Corporate entities can now pay unlimited amounts of money to political action groups (super PACs) to indirectly finance politicians' campaigns. They can also lobby politicians either to pass legislation that will advance their corporate interests or, alternatively, to block legislation that seeks to regulate or tax them. In like manner, big money controls health care. The AMA lobbies on behalf of doctors; the AHA on behalf of hospitals; and many other health care related entities, such as insurers, pharmaceutical companies and device makers, have their lobbies as well.

Since the earliest days of our Republic, government has always been about the balancing of two conflicting forces: the rights of each of us as individuals, and the health and welfare of all of the members of our society; the struggle between our own self-interest on the one hand, and the public interest and social progress on the other. Most of us would like to demand the most for ourselves, but are properly constrained by both our personal morality and the laws of our country.

In the aftermath of World War II, the United States stood as a constructive and democratic model for the world. We helped rebuild Europe. We grew a broad middle class of workers, teachers, business owners, doctors and lawyers, and passed civil rights legislation as well as Medicare and Medicaid. We had a broad expanding productive middle class in manufacturing, construction, services and farming. Government programs like social security, Medicare and Medicaid provided the old and poor with a safety net. Public education was generally good and was supported by local governments as well as by the Federal government. Medical care was mostly available at affordable prices.

President Dwight Eisenhower warned us about the "military-industrial complex" taking control of America back in the 1950s. I remember. He was talking about the cozy and ultimately mutually lucrative relationships between government officials in departments charged with establishing military policy and corporations supplying military equipment and services. Eisenhower must be turning over in his grave now. These "complexes" of government policy makers and private corporations have subsumed every area of our economy. He could probably never even have envisioned the deadly behemoth of the financial services industry that controls so much of our economy. This is an industry that to a large extent produces no useful product, just wealth for itself, and simply drains resources from the rest of us.

Starting in the 1980s, something basic to our values as a society in America changed. As a country, we were no longer the altruistic heroes of the world as we had been following World War II. As we became a more individually self-interested and unregulated capitalistic society, many new millionaires and billionaires emerged. The vibrant middle class began disappearing in America and continues to do so today. Greed became good; the public interest less important.

Unions, a powerful bulwark for the middle class earlier, became less popular politically and socially as corporate power increased. Granted, some unions had become corrupted and over-empowered in some ways, ultimately weakening themselves. But unions in general, then and now, have been the single most important force counterbalancing ruthless self-interest of employers, especially in the private industrial sector. Ronald Reagan helped union busting by firing air traffic controllers as one of his first acts in the early '80s. Lobbyists for the large corporations became much more abundant and have mushroomed to their current major prominence in crafting policy and enacting the laws of the land today. This political influence on public policy has reached an intolerable point of government catering mainly to the wishes of the rich and powerful.

Many Americans have become hypnotized by a conservative narrative portraying America as the land where anyone who works hard enough and wants to succeed badly enough can make it to the top. The Horatio Alger success myth suggests that anyone from any strata of American society can achieve great success, and that those who cannot become self-sufficient are "slackers." In this view, there is little or no need for safety nets or government regulation or reasonably high taxes on millionaires. The Horatio Alger myth is still realized today by some people who "pull themselves up by their bootstraps," as the saying goes, but these people are proportionately very few in number and they are usually sports figures and entertainers along with a few successful entrepreneurs. Much more often, people succeed when they are born into well-to-do families, and fail when they belong to poorer ones, despite their best efforts. The well-to-do get a better education and more job opportunities. Studies have shown that over the past 30 years it has been increasingly more difficult for Americans to exit the poorer class, and enter the middle class (NYT). And, in fact, the wages of the average American worker have been stagnant and level over this time.

As is detailed so well in Thomas Frank's book, "What's the Matter with Kansas," politicians have exploited religious affiliations, racial intolerance, anti-abortion positions and anti-gay biases, to persuade middle America to elect anti-government conservatives to Congress. These elected politicians who purport to represent the middle class then turn around and vote for policies favoring the rich, and against policies involving government programs which would benefit the middle class, thus acting contrary to the self-interest of the people they persuaded to vote for them in the first place.

In 1933, the Glass-Steagall Act was passed, preventing the co-mingling of the activities of commercial and investment banks that led to the financial abuses resulting in the Great Depression. In 1999, the ultimate triumph of the powerful financial sector was the repeal of this Act, which led to the merging of the activities of commercial banks and investment banks, and, eventually, to the financial meltdown in our economy in 2008. New entities like credit default swaps and derivatives were created and traded by the big banks and financial institutions and generated huge profits. Subprime mortgage lending and the dicing and bundling of mortgages into so-called mortgage-backed securities and the selling and re-selling of these securities were also heavily promoted and hugely profitable for the banks. These high-risk transactions were akin to the unregulated activities of huge gambling casinos. And it all began, it should be noted, in the late '90s, overseen by a Democratic president, Bill Clinton, and his financial team led by Robert Rubin, the Treasury secretary.

Then came the disastrous policies of the Bush-Cheney administration. The tax benefits to the rich and the expenses of two wars which were paid for with borrowed money were the final death knell blows to our economic well-being. In addition to the financial meltdown of 2008, our current huge deficit situation and the unemployment crisis that exists today, are the legacies of these disastrous policies.

Many of us, both liberals and true conservatives alike, are really mad not only about the bailouts of the financial industry, but also about the continuing lack of accountability of the financial industry as we struggle to emerge from our recent recession. Enormous government support in the form of these bailouts and low interest rates has saved the day for the very same right-wing conservatives who hate big government, except when it benefits them. The big banks and the financial industry are today back to their pre-recession profit-making levels and CEO salaries are higher than ever. At the same time, no significant government benefits have been given to the millions of Americans who, as a result of the housing recession and mortgage fiascos, went underwater and/or became bankrupt because of their mortgages. The double whammy of mortgage debt and unemployment has left the American economy in tatters.

And most recently, the Supreme Court, now dominated by so-called conservative justices (so-called because no Supreme Court has been more activist and dismissive of precedents), has increased the power and influence of the rich and powerful further by allowing any individual, corporation or interest group to spend as much money in political campaigns as it wishes without restriction.

Perhaps the greatest problem of all is that we, the American public, are poorly informed and inadequately concerned about the power of special interests to control our lives, mainly through the political process. Despite the extraordinary expansion of sources of information available to us, especially the Internet and social media as well as the printed press, radio and television, we as a society have become much more focused on our own self-interest as individuals than on our responsibilities as citizens. Who has time to think about and respond to the disasters generated by special interests that are occurring in our society as a whole: financial chaos, unemployment; inefficient and expensive health care; declining public education; infrastructure deterioration; environmental pollution? Instead, we are totally absorbed in just keeping ourselves financially afloat while at the same time keeping up with all the ways our gadgets, iPhones and iPads with all their apps and games, and Facebook, Twitter and YouTube can entertain us and fill our days.

We all got along reasonably well when we interacted more personally and directly with each other through conversations, and so did our elected representatives who used to be able to cooperate with each other in crafting legislation for everyone's benefit. But that was in a once upon a time that we may not soon, if ever, see again.

Increased government debt has led to the loss of millions of government jobs at the federal and state levels. There have been massive layoffs of teachers, fire fighters and police officers, the core pillars of our society. The American economy as a whole, and our work force in particular, has benefited incredibly little from our increased enmeshment in the global economy. We, as a society, have done nothing to protect American jobs from leaving the United States and going to emerging powerhouses with lower wages like India and China.

As a matter of societal policy, this is intolerable. Apple Computer, an American company born and bred, and now the most successful company in the world, has most of its jobs overseas, benefiting mainly China. I am a huge Apple user, and I enjoy the relatively low price of their products, but I am beginning to feel like a traitor to my country as I continue to use these products. I would be willing to pay more for them if that is the price of keeping jobs in the United States. There should be financial consequences to Apple and other American companies for the outsourcing of jobs. I believe in "Made in the USA" as much as possible. Either higher taxes or high tariffs for their products should be the price for American companies that outsource their jobs.

Jeffrey Immelt, CEO of General Electric, and recently (and to my mind, without reason) the head of President Obama's Jobs Council, was on CBS's 60 minutes in 2011. In his interview, he seemed unabashedly proud when he stated that he felt that his primary obligation as CEO of GE was "to my investors," not to the best interests of the United States. He indicated that he spent most of his time as CEO finding places other than the US that were better suited to invest in because these foreign investments would better bolster GE's bottom line. There was no mention of the need for the United States to prosper financially or any obligation to help create jobs in the United States.

Many young people, seeing the personal economic success of individuals working in the financial industry, have entered the financial services field in the past two decades in the hope of becoming rich quickly, and some have succeeded. More recently, with some contraction of the financial industry, this has become a less desirable career path. At the same time, other employment possibilities have withered away as the economy has suffered in terms of housing, manufacturing jobs, and federal and state employment opportunities. People, particularly young people, have begun recognizing the problems of the increasing gap between the parasitically rich and everybody else and supporting movements in the opposite direction, like Occupy Wall Street. Although I, and many others, feel that this is a positive development, it must be accompanied by political action to have an effective impact on our society. The stakes are high. Extreme inequality of wealth translates into extreme inequality of opportunity and the death of meritocracy, the very heart of the spectacular American success story.

We all want to make enough money to feel comfortable financially. I certainly have tried to earn as much as I could during my career. But I, along with most people, would rather do more than just make money. I think people need to feel useful in society, to have jobs they experience as being intrinsically valuable. I think traditional bankers and traders and brokers who, by working with money, help people build their businesses and find financial security have a very legitimate place in our society and a real societal purpose. I think this is also true of bankers who facilitate sales, acquisitions, and mergers of businesses. But I don't think this is true of many other people in the large Wall Street firms, and the banking and financial services industries today. They have helped rig the world's financial markets only to maximize their own profits, and have manipulated and destroyed much of America's wealth as well as that of many other developed nations around the world that have followed the high-risk and dubious practices of American financiers.

America Divided

Most Americans want to make a comfortable living and live a normal middle class life while doing what they like, whether working with their hands or heads or both; in construction, running a business, providing services, or being in a profession like medicine, law, teaching, the clergy. Or if they are particularly talented, working in the arts or sports or entertainment. Doing something personally rewarding that provides enough money to live comfortably and to be free from financial anxieties. But today, wealth is the principal goal and often the only goal of too many, and what used to be on the highest rung of personal and societal values — achievement benefiting community, family enriching integrity, and religious or non-religious concern with social welfare — are all secondary. A profound divide has developed between those who care about the health and welfare and success of their fellow Americans, and those who think principally about becoming wealthy and benefiting only themselves.

With respect to our views of medical care, Americans are again divided along the same general battle lines: those who think that medical care is a universal right of all of its citizens, and those who think that their rights as individuals supersede the needs of the other members of our society. I think the difference between these two groups is the difference between members of a civilized society on one hand, and cold unfeeling individualists on the other.

While we work on solutions to our problems of universal and efficient and affordable medical care and insurance, we must also solve our crises in public education, job creation, deteriorating infrastructure and environmental protection. Government and the private sector must work together on all of these issues, all of which impact our health as a country. The public school system in the United States made my enjoyment of my life and work possible. I don't know the precise reasons for the deterioration of the system and the poor showing of academic skills by American students vis à vis students in other countries, but I know that it is absolutely vital that we train and support excellent teachers and excellent schools if our society is to successfully compete and flourish in the future.

Teachers must be paid well. Schools must be repaired or replaced. I know this is being talked about both locally and in Washington, but the results so far have been another political stand-off. The conservatives don't want to spend the money or raise taxes either locally or nationally to support higher teacher pay and better education for all. And many of our citizens think paying for cable television and smart phones is much more important than paying more in taxes to support their local public schools. This mindset must be changed.

In our approach to all of our problems relating to financial inequality, the deterioration of public education, the health care crisis, the degradation of our environment, our woefully inadequate gun laws, and our crumbling infrastructure in the United States, we face a fundamental question: How much do we care about our own self-interest versus how important is it to us that our American society as a whole prospers and enriches the lives of all of our citizens, who, in turn, would then be able to fulfill their potential and further enrich our society as a whole?

CHAPTER NINETEEN

The Last Chapter

There is no predictable chapter, especially no predictable last chapter, in any of our lives. This undercurrent of uncertainty has its good and bad aspects. We feel that we have at least some measure of free will at any given moment in our lives to determine what we do, while simultaneously we know that at any given moment we can lose that control and have a heart attack or get cancer or get run over by a bus. Or lose our jobs and our homes. Luck, serendipity, is a major player even though we would all like to believe that we are largely masters of our own fate.

In my case, I know I was fortunate to be born with certain abilities, and to be born in the USA into a household that met my basic needs, and into a community that provided me with fine educational opportunities. These were gifts from the cosmos. Nothing I did made them happen. I was just lucky.

I had the good fortune to be able to use what I had learned from excellent teachers in well-run schools to move forward with my life and eventually enter a profession. None of these events were pre-determined or even primarily influenced by me. I take little credit for them. So when, in my musings, I think of myself as an American self-made man, rising from some lower level by "pulling myself up by my bootstraps," as many would have me believe, I know this is not really true. It was mainly serendipity. I was born in the right place at the right time. I went to the right schools and had the right teachers, and that is all it really took for me to achieve my own personal success. Yes, I worked hard and did well, but if I had been born into other circumstances that did not provide those same supports and opportunities, all of my work would have been for naught.

America gave me all I needed to become me. I grew up in a mid-twentieth century America of educational and professional opportunities for which I will forever be grateful. But as I grew up, I also became aware that many people of different ethnicities were largely excluded from these opportunities and this awareness has been fundamental to my life-long political support of leaders committed to seeing that young people of all races and socio-economic backgrounds have access to as many paths to realizing their potential as I did. I am willing to pay as much in taxes as is necessary to have America prosper, and especially to support public education. I would like to think that I have given back something of value to our society through my work as a physician and scientist as well as my actions as a citizen, but I feel that I have not given nearly as much to America as America has given to me.

America is struggling today to keep alive the American dream for all of its children. But there is more poverty and income inequality in America than I have ever seen before. The public school system is not as effective in meeting the educational demands of the day as it was when I was growing up, and the financial challenges of obtaining quality higher education and professional opportunities are much more daunting than those that I was able, with determination and work, to meet. It is a national tragedy that our great public as well as private universities have become out of the financial reach of so many high school graduates all across the country. This must change if America is to move forward in an increasingly competitive world.

I was able to become a physician and scientist, doing work I loved and enjoyed, and I have lived a fulfilling life. I have amassed no great wealth, but have done well enough, and now live comfortably in retirement. I would have liked to have lived a less stressful life, not as pressed, especially in my growing up years, to make money, but overall, I can't complain. I have largely done only what I wanted to do, with few bosses or restrictions. Not many people can say that.

What has been the core of my being? What has driven me? What have been my goals? They have been largely the same as everyone else's: to be free and independent; to fall in love; to have enough money to afford a decent life for both myself and my family; to have a good job. I have never had any high ideals or great goals for myself except to survive, to love my wife and family, to have a career that intrinsically excited me. I never wanted to sacrifice any more of my freedom and independence than absolutely necessary for financial security, although I have always craved that security. I chose a career mostly in medical research over one primarily in clinical medicine because I loved it. I could have made a lot more money in the private practice of clinical medicine and hematology-oncology, but I wanted to do laboratory research primarily so I became a research physician and an academic clinician.

I was always excited and enthusiastic about all of my professional activities: research, clinical care and teaching; and I always tried my best to transmit that excitement and enthusiasm to others. I thought I would continue doing research, treating people and teaching until the day I died. However, around the year 2000 and near my 65th birthday, I began to feel professionally burned out. I was surprised by my emotional letdown at work, but I just didn't have that extra zeal I had always had before. It became harder for me to be as completely involved and focused on all aspects of my professional responsibilities, and I began to feel resentful of all the pressures on me at work. I just didn't have the same enthusiasm and intensity that had characterized my professional life until then, and which I believe are required for professional success at a high level.

The first major change I made was to curtail some of my clinical activities. I gave up making medical ward rounds and attending hematology outpatient clinic. That eased my workload somewhat. Then, in 2002, in the midst of doing what I thought was my most exciting NIH funded research on human globin gene regulation, my research grant in this area was not renewed. That event became a tipping point. I no longer had the funds to run as big a lab as I felt I needed to continue to pursue my research projects in globin gene regulation as well as in human globin gene therapy, the other field in which I also had had long term NIH funded research success. I struggled along.

In 2005, Columbia University offered its older professors like me a very attractive retirement plan. I didn't have to think about it long. I took it. As it happened, I had put in a new grant to continue to work on human globin gene therapy that same year. That grant was funded, and so, transitioning from full-time full speed ahead academia to semi-retirement, I continued to work part-time at Columbia on experiments to devise new ways to perform human globin gene therapy for sickle cell disease and thalassemia. We made progress with this grant in developing new technology to facilitate the transfer of normal human hemoglobin genes into human cells, but it was not the immediately useful clinical breakthrough that I had hoped for. Funding for this research ended in 2009. I continued to give lectures to medical students at Columbia on human gene therapy until stopping for good in 2011.

Since leaving Columbia University, I have continued my life-long habit of doing odd jobs, which in recent decades had taken the form of consulting for lawyers and for biotech companies. I also keep up with the literature in the fields of my interest today. I continue to be a member of the American Society of Hematology (ASH) and read its publication, the journal Blood. I had been going to the annual meeting of ASH almost every year since 1964, often as a contributor to the annual meeting, submitting abstracts and/or presenting papers most years, and I had published many research papers and review articles in Blood as well. But I have recently stopped.

I certainly don't miss the turmoil of scientific life either inside or outside the lab. Doing science at a high level is a contact sport. The competition for grants is fierce and getting papers published in the best journals is always a hassle. However, I am still excited and interested when I read about new findings by my former competitors and others in the fields of my interest.

Today, as a retiree, I am happy as long as I can get a good night's sleep, have a good swim, enjoy a good breakfast, and read The New York Times. I live with my wife in an apartment in Riverdale, the Bronx, overlooking the Hudson River with a straight-on view of the Palisades, a view of which I never tire. I continue to be a New York sports fan: a Knicks fan, a Mets fan and a Giants football fan; a ballet enthusiast, a movie and show patron, a mystery and history book reader, and a weekly poker player. I believe in and contribute to MoveOn.org. I also continue to give medical advice to anyone who asks me because I don't think my medical judgment has deteriorated significantly over time. Of course, I don't treat anybody and when I think medical attention is called for, I refer my "patients" to the best doctors I know.

Finally, in the last eight years, I have experienced the special joy of being a grandparent. My wish for my grandchildren and for all the children and grandchildren of our beloved country is a better America of equal educational and employment opportunities, a true meritocracy of more equitable wealth distribution, with food, housing, and health care security for all.

About the Author

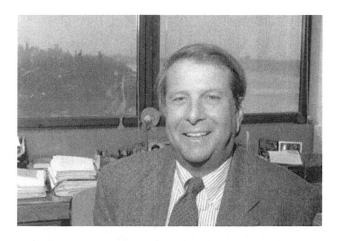

Arthur Bank, M.D. has been a scientist, clinician and teacher at Columbia University and Presbyterian Hospital for over 40 years, and was Head of the Division of Hematology at Columbia-Presbyterian Medical Center. An international leader in the field of hematology research, he has published extensively on the mechanisms of human globin gene regulation and human gene therapy, and is the author of *Turning Blood Red: The Fight for Life in Cooley's Anemia* (2009). Dr. Bank is currently Professor Emeritus of Medicine and of Genetics and Development at Columbia University.

Index